100 Questions & Answers About Lymphoma

Peter Holman, MD
Jodi Garrett, RN
William D. Jansen

JONES AND BARTLETT PUBLISHERS
Sudbury, Massachusetts
BOSTON   TORONTO   LONDON   SINGAPORE

World Headquarters
Jones and Bartlett
Publishers
40 Tall Pine Drive
Sudbury, MA 01776
info@jbpub.com
www.jbpub.com

Jones and Bartlett
Publishers Canada
2406 Nikanna Road
Mississauga, ON L5C
2W6
CANADA

Jones and Bartlett
Publishers International
Barb House, Barb Mews
London W6 7PA
UK

Library of Congress Cataloging-in-Publication Data

Holman, Peter, M.D.
　100 questions & answers about lymphoma / Peter Holman, Jodi Garett,
William D. Jansen.
　　p. cm.
　ISBN 0-7637-2039-9
　1. Lymphomas--Popular works.　2. Lymphomas--Miscellanea.　I. Title:
One hundred questions and answers about lymphoma.　II. Garrett, Jodi.
III. Jansen, William D.　IV. Title.
　RC280.L9H65　2003
　616.99'446--dc21

　　　　　　　　　　　　　　　　　　　　　　2003000517

The authors, editor, and publisher have made every effort to provide accurate information. However, they are not responsible for errors, omissions, or for any outcomes related to the use of the contents of this book and take no responsibility for the use of the products described. Treatments and side effects described in this book may not be applicable to all patients; likewise, some patients may require a dose or experience a side effect that is not described herein. The reader should confer with his or her own physician regarding specific treatments and side effects. Drugs and medical devices are discussed that may have limited availability controlled by the Food and Drug Administration (FDA) for use only in a research study or clinical trial. The drug information presented has been derived from reference sources, recently published data, and pharmaceutical research data. Research, clinical practice, and government regulations often change the accepted standard in this field. When consideration is being given to use of any drug in the clinical setting, the healthcare provider or reader is responsible for determining FDA status of the drug, reading the package insert, reviewing prescribing information for the most up-to-date recommendations on dose, precautions, and contraindications, and determining the appropriate usage for the product. This is especially important in the case of drugs that are new or seldom used.

Acquisitions Editor: Christopher Davis
Production Editor: Elizabeth Platt
Cover Design: Philip Regan
Manufacturing Buyer: Therese Bräuer
Composition: Northeast Compositors
Printing and Binding: Malloy Lithographing
Cover Printer: Malloy Lithographing

Printed in the United States of America

07 06 05 04　　　10 9 8 7 6 5 4 3 2

Contents

Questions 1–10 introduce the immune and circulatory systems, describing their function and involvement in lymphoma through such questions as:

- What is the immune system?
- How do the components of the immune system function?
- What are lymphocytes?
- How does the immune system fight infection?
- How is the immune system important in lymphoma?

Questions 11–22 briefly outline the different types of lymphoma and describe their diagnosis and classification, including:

- What is lymphoma? What is Hodgkin's disease? What is non-Hodgkin's lymphoma?
- What are the symptoms of lymphoma?
- How is lymphoma diagnosed?
- How is a bone marrow examination performed?

Questions 23–44 provide a more detailed account of different types of lymphoma and the methods by which they are differentiated, including:

- What type of lymphoma do I have?
- What are the different types of Hodgkin's disease?
- Can Hodgkin's disease turn into non-Hodgkin's lymphoma?

Questions 45–57 discuss treatment options for various forms of lymphoma, including:

- What happens after I'm told that I have lymphoma?
- What is the IPI?

According to the American Cancer Society, approximately 61,000 new cases of lymphoma will be diagnosed in the United States in 2003. Of these, approximately 53,400 cases will be non-Hodgkin's lymphoma, and the remaining cases (7,600) will be Hodgkin's disease. Since the early 1970s, for unclear reasons, the incidence of lymphoma has doubled and continues to rise.

The term "lymphoma" actually describes many different but related diseases. Although there is overlap, the different lymphomas tend to affect people in different ways. There are even some types of lymphoma that may not always require treatment; for most lymphomas, however, there are a number of treatment choices that can be made in any particular situation. It is therefore a major challenge for individuals receiving such a diagnosis to obtain the relevant information necessary to be an active participant in their care. The Internet is a very useful source of information, but it also contains much disinformation that can be more damaging and frightening than helpful.

In this book, written for patients and their caregivers, we (a physician, a nurse, and a patient) have attempted to provide an understanding of lymphoma—both non-Hodgkin's lymphoma and Hodgkin's disease—that will assist you in understanding this disease and coping with the daily pressures of the fight against lymphoma. In addition, the Appendix includes links to sites with additional information about lymphoma-related clinical research and clinical trials. We hope you find it useful.

Peter Holman, MD
Jodi Garrett, RN
William D. Jansen

PART ONE

The Basics: Understanding the Immune and Circulatory Systems

What is the immune system?

How do the components of the immune system function?

More ...

1. What is the immune system?

Your body's **immune system** protects you from illnesses by eliminating dangerous foreign (abnormal) substances. This system is your main defense against all infections (illness arising from invasion from an outside organism, such as bacteria or viruses) and also plays an important role in how your body responds to many diseases, including lymphoma and other cancers. Individuals in whom the immune system is not functioning properly have an increased risk of certain cancers (including lymphoma), as well as a much higher risk of many types of infection.

The immune system has a variety of important components, including a circulation system of **lymphatic channels** that connects the **lymph nodes** or **lymph glands**, the **tonsils**, the **spleen**, and the **thymus** (Figure 1). The spleen essentially functions like a very large lymph node and is located in the abdomen below the left lung. The thymus is an organ that is located behind the breastbone (sternum) in children and young adults; it becomes inactive in older adults. The circulating **lymph fluid** contains large numbers of **lymphocytes**—white blood cells that fight disease. The lymphocytes are the "foot soldiers" of the immune system, directly responsible for destroying invading organisms or disease cells.

The two main types of lymphocytes (**B cells** and **T cells**) act together with other immune cells to mount an attack in response to foreign invaders such as infections. The manner in which disease cells are recognized is essential in the body's success or failure in fending off an illness. For example, under certain circumstances,

---

Immune system

the complex system by which the body protects itself from outside invaders that are harmful.

Lymphatic channels

the tiny vessels that connect the lymph glands.

Lymph nodes

another term for lymph glands.

Lymph glands

the large collections of lymphocytes present at intervals throughout the lymph system. They can get big and painful in response to an infection.

Tonsils

large lymph nodes present in the back of the throat.

Spleen

the large lymph-node–like organ under the lower left ribs.

Thymus

an organ behind the breast bone that is important for the development of an immune response, especially in children.

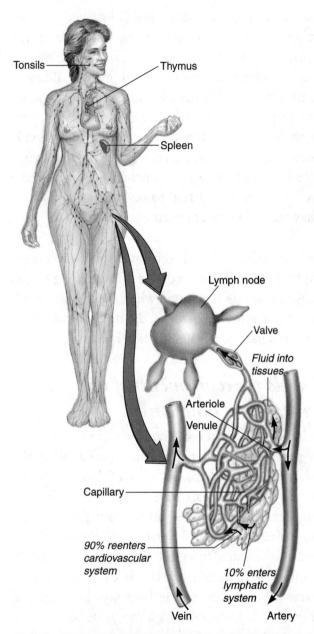

Tonsils

Thymus

Spleen

Lymph node

Valve

Fluid into tissues

Arteriole

Venule

Capillary

90% reenters cardiovascular system

10% enters lymphatic system

Vein

Artery

Figure 1   The lymphatic system consists of the lymphatic vessels and ducts, lymph nodes (which are distributed throughout the body), the tonsils, the thymus gland, and the spleen. The enlarged diagram of a lymph node and vessels shows the path of the excess fluid that leaves the arteriole end of a capillary bed, enters the adjacent tissue spaces, and is absorbed by lymphatic capillaries. Reprinted from Alters S: *Biology: Understanding Life*, Third Ed. Copyright ©1999 Jones and Bartlett Publishers, Inc.

Lymph fluid

the fluid that carries lymphocytes around the body.

Lymphocytes

the main type of cell that makes up the immune system and is the abnormal cell in lymphoma.

B cells

a type of lymphocyte.

T cells

one of the major types of lymphocytes.

Autoimmune disease

an illness in which a person's own immune system regards parts of its own body as foreign.

lymphocytes mistake an individual's own body tissues for foreign substances. In such cases, this error results in an immune attack on normal tissues; such attacks are called an **autoimmune disease** and include illnesses such as rheumatoid arthritis and systemic lupus erythematosus. Importantly, in most cancers, including lymphoma, the immune system fails in the opposite way: It does not recognize the cancer cells as foreign and therefore allows the cancer to grow unchecked. Clearly, the ability of the immune system to respond appropriately is one key factor in cancer treatment.

The body initially "trains" T cells to distinguish foreign proteins from normal body proteins. This training occurs in the thymus during childhood when the thymus is still an active organ; after adolescence, the thymus shrinks (or involutes) and has little or no function in adults.

2. How do the components of the immune system function?

Two circulatory systems transport immune cells around the body. Most people are familiar with the blood circulatory system, in which blood cells are transported from the heart to the lungs to obtain oxygen and then via the arteries throughout the body. Its job is to deliver oxygen and nutrients to the body's tissues and at the same time get rid of carbon dioxide, waste, and toxic matter from the body. These wastes and toxins are removed in the liver and kidneys, and carbon dioxide is transported via the veins back to the lungs, where it is exchanged for more oxygen. In addition to this function of supplying oxygen and removing waste substances, the blood also carries disease- and injury-fighting **white blood cells**, which include the lymphocytes and a number of other cells (described in Questions 4 and 6), and many other types of protein that are important for blood clotting.

Most of us, however, have only a small understanding of the lymphatic circulatory system, which works alongside the blood circulatory system in fighting disease. The lymphatic circulation system transports the lymph fluid containing the lymphocytes around the body in lymph channels in much the same way as blood is transported via arteries and veins. Lymphocytes are first produced in the **bone marrow** (see Question 3), after which they travel through both the bloodstream and lymphatic channels to the lymph nodes and/or the thymus (in children) and then back into the bloodstream. The lymphatic channels that comprise the lymphatic circulatory system consist of tiny, thin, leaky vessels that carry lymph fluid back toward the heart. They usually run alongside the veins, which likewise carry blood back to the heart from various parts of the body.

At frequent intervals along the lymphatic channels, large clusters of lymphocytes occur. These are the lymph nodes or glands in which lymphocytes often first encounter a foreign protein or **antigen**. When a lymphocyte recognizes a protein as foreign, it sends out signals to other lymphocytes that it needs help to mount an immune response that will get rid of the foreign protein. Lymphocytes increase in the region, and when they are activated through their encounter with the foreign substance, they secrete chemical messengers that arrange the appropriate immune response. If

White blood cells
blood cells that are most important for fighting infection.

The Basics

Bone marrow
the liquid inside part of bone where the blood cells are produced.

Antigen
any substance that can induce an immune response. This could be an infection or a cancer cell.

you've ever had red, swollen tonsils (which are lymphatic organs in the throat) during an infection or a cold, then you've experienced this firsthand. Because of the increase of lymphocytes, it is not unusual for lymph nodes, tonsils, and sometimes even the spleen to become enlarged and painful during a serious infection. This accumulation reflects the immune system's attempt to control and eliminate the infection. Lymph nodes occur throughout the body but, when enlarged, they are most easily felt in the neck, armpits, and groin. Collections of nodes also occur in the chest, between the lungs, and in the abdomen, where they are found beside the **aorta** and the **inferior vena cava**, which runs alongside the aorta and carries blood back from your legs and abdomen to your heart.

The spleen is a specialized part of the immune system that functions as a very large lymph node. It is about the size of your fist and sits below your left lung under the ribs. The spleen is essentially a very large collection of lymphocytes and is another site where lymphocytes come into contact with foreign proteins. Certain infections, including infectious mononucleosis (commonly called glandular fever) and malaria, can result in an enlarged spleen. When this occurs, your physician can sometimes feel the spleen (if it is normal size, it cannot be felt) in your abdomen. Under certain circumstances, the spleen needs to be surgically removed. If this is necessary, especially in children, antibiotics may be prescribed to prevent certain types of infection. Although you can live a normal life without a spleen, it is an important part of the immune system, providing significant protection against some types of infection; thus, patients without a spleen should seek medical attention quickly in the event of an infection.

Aorta

the main blood vessel (artery) that carries blood from the heart to the smaller arteries delivering blood to all parts of the body.

Inferior vena cava

the large vein that carries blood back toward the heart.

You can think of these components as a defensive army that is fighting a continuing battle against would-be invaders. The lymphocyte "ground troops" are armed within the bone marrow (during childhood, they are also sent out for "training" in the thymus). Then they patrol the body via the lymphatic system and encounter invaders and battle in the nodes and, during cases of very serious invasion, in the tonsils and spleen as well.

3. What is bone marrow?

The bone marrow is the soft substance that is present inside many of the bones in your body. It is where all blood cells are produced and contains the blood-forming **stem cells**, which can produce **red blood cells**, white blood cells, and **platelets**. All of these cells go though a number of different stages of maturation in the bone marrow before they are ready to be released into the bloodstream. If the bloodstream becomes deficient in any type of cell, such as a low red blood cell count in a patient with **anemia**, the bone marrow can attempt to replace the missing red blood cells by increasing production. Bone marrow is present in the skull, backbone (vertebrae), ribs, hip, or pelvic bones and at the top ends of the **humerus** (upper arm bone) and **femur** (thigh bone). Normally, fat cells take up approximately half the bone marrow space; the other half consists of the blood-forming cells.

4. What are lymphocytes?

Lymphocytes are one type of white blood cell (other white blood cells are described in Question 6; see Figure 2). Although they too fight disease, lymphocytes are the "foot soldiers" of the immune system, and it is

You can think of these components as a defensive army that is fighting a continuing battle against would-be invaders.

The Basics

Stem cells
the cells that can produce red cells, white cells, and platelets.

Red blood cells
the most common type of blood cells that carry oxygen around the body.

Platelets
the tiny blood cells that are produced in the bone marrow and are important for blood clotting.

Anemia
a low hemoglobin level.

Humerus
the major bone connecting the shoulder to the elbow.

Femur
the thigh bone.

	BLOOD CELL TYPE	DESCRIPTION	FUNCTION	LIFE SPAN
RED BLOOD CELLS	Erythrocyte	Flat disk with a central depression, no nucleus, contain hemoglobin.	Transport oxygen (O_2) and carbon dioxide (CO_2).	About 120 days.
WHITE BLOOD CELLS (LEUKOCYTES) — Granulocytes	Neutrophil	Spherical; with many lobed nucleus, no hemoglobin, pink-purple **cytoplasmic granules.**	Cellular defense-phagocytosis of small microorganisms.	Hours to 3 days.
	Eosinophil	Spherical; two-lobed nucleus, no hemoglobin, orange-red staining **cytoplasmic granules.**	Cellular defense- phagocytosis of large microorganisms such as parasitic worms, releases anti-inflammatory substances in allergic reactions.	8 to 12 days.
	Basophil	Spherical; generally two-lobed nucleus, no hemoglobin large purple staining **cytoplasmic granules.**	Inflammatory response - contain granules that rupture and release chemicals enhancing inflammatory response.	Hours to 3 days.
Agranulocytes	Monocyte	Spherical; **single nucleus** shaped like kidney bean, no cytoplasmic granules, cytoplasm often blue in color.	Converted to macrophage which are large cells that entrap microorganisms and other foreign matter.	Days to months.
	B-lymphocyte	Spherical; round **singular nucleus**, no cytoplasmic granules.	Immune system response and regulation, antibody production sometimes cause allergic response.	Days to years.
	T-lymphocyte	Spherical; round **singular nucleus**, no cytoplasmic granules.	Immune system response and regulation; cellular immune response.	Days to years.
PLATELETS	Platelets	Irregularly shaped fragments, very small pink staining granules.	Control blood clotting or coagulation.	7 to 10 days.

Figure 2   Types of blood cells. Reprinted from Alters S: *Biology: Understanding Life*, Third Ed. Copyright ©1999 Jones and Bartlett Publishers, Inc.

specifically these cells that lymphoma affects (Question 1). The two main types of lymphocytes, B and T cells, have different roles in working to eliminate foreign proteins (antigens) from the body, but they work together to achieve the same result of preventing and eliminating illnesses.

B lymphocytes are named for where they come from in chicken embryos—an organ called the "bursa of Fabricious," although humans have no such organ and our bone marrow manufactures B cells (the name has stuck simply because it's a convenient identifier). T cells are so called because of the important role that the thymus plays in their development.

As with B cells, T lymphocytes are produced in your bone marrow. From here, they circulate throughout the body using both blood vessels and lymphatic channels. T and B cells look identical when blood is examined under a microscope, but the types of molecules or protein substances on their surface can help to distinguish them. Specialized laboratory equipment found in most hospitals or clinical laboratories can be used to distinguish the different types of lymphocytes on the basis of these proteins. It is the growth and accumulation of large numbers of lymphocytes that result in the lymph node enlargement that occurs in lymphoma.

5. What are the other types of blood cells?

In addition to lymphocytes, the bone marrow produces many other types of blood cells (Figure 2) that are the offspring of one very important bone marrow cell called the **hematopoietic stem cell**, which gets it name because it can produce all of the blood cells ("hematopoietic" is derived from the Greek words *haimatos*, which means blood, and *poiein*, which means to make). Embryonic stem cells, the subject of much ongoing scientific, ethical, and political discussion, differ from these cells, as they can give rise to cells of many more different tissues than the hematopoietic stem cell. Thus, when stem cells are discussed in this context, we mean strictly the hematopoietic stem cells that give rise *only* to blood cells.

Hematopoietic stem cell

the most immature cell that develops into red cells, white blood cells, and platelets.

The main groups of blood cells are red cells, white cells, and platelets. As mentioned previously here, the B and T lymphocytes are only two of a number of different types of white blood cells (Question 6).

6. What are the other types of white cells?

All of the white cells are produced in the bone marrow. They make their way into the bloodstream where they circulate for a varying length of time before moving into the tissues of the body. They can carry out their functions in the bloodstream or various tissues.

Neutrophils are the most common type of white blood cells, with lymphocytes second. Neutrophils are easily identified under a microscope as having a **nucleus** that is divided up into three or four lobes. The **cytoplasm** (the part of the cell that surrounds the nucleus) of the neutrophils contains **granules**, which in turn contain chemicals (**enzymes**) that are important for killing bacteria. When someone has a bacterial infection, the number of white cells in the blood normally increases, mostly because of an increase in neutrophils.

Chemotherapy, which is a name for medications used to treat disease—cancer, in this case—can be used to kill the cancer cells, but it also prevents the bone marrow's production of neutrophils. People receiving chemotherapy therefore have periods when they are at an increased risk of infection from bacteria. For this reason, many patients on chemotherapy also receive **growth factors**, which increase the neutrophil count, or antibiotics to prevent an infection.

Other white blood cells include monocytes, eosinophils, and basophils. The monocytes are also important in pre-

Neutrophils

the main white blood cell important for fighting infection.

Nucleus

the central part of the cell that contains the genetic information.

Cytoplasm

the part of a cell that surrounds the central nucleus.

Granules

small particles containing enzymes.

Enzymes

chemical messengers within the body.

Chemotherapy

treating a disease with drugs; usually refers to the different types of drugs used to treat cancer.

Growth factors

chemicals that can be injected to stimulate the production of blood cells.

venting and controlling bacterial infections. Eosinophils are important in responding to parasites and have a role in allergic reactions. The white blood cell count is usually normal in people when they are diagnosed with lymphoma, but it is important to know which types of white blood cells are present in the blood, as even when the white blood cell count is normal, lymphoma cells can be found circulating in the blood.

7. What are red blood cells?

Red blood cells, the most common type of blood cells, do not have a nucleus but contain a red pigment called **hemoglobin**, which is essential to life because it allows oxygen to be carried around the body. The hemoglobin level determines whether someone has anemia, which is easily established by performing a **complete blood count (CBC)**. The most common reasons for people with lymphoma to develop anemia are the presence of lymphoma in the bone marrow or the effect of chemotherapy on the bone marrow cells that produce the red blood cells.

8. What are platelets?

Large cells called **megakaryocytes**, make platelets (the smallest type of blood cell) in the bone marrow. Platelets are very important in preventing and healing bleeding and bruising. Your platelets may be low because lymphoma in the bone marrow can affect the megakaryocytes' production of platelets or because of chemotherapy. Rarely, platelet counts of lymphoma patients can be low because their lymphocytes produce **antibodies** that can attach to their platelets. The

The Basics

Hemoglobin

a protein present in red blood cells that carries oxygen.

Complete blood count

a blood test looking at the red cell count, the hemoglobin, the white count, and the platelet count.

Megakaryocytes

the bone marrow cells that produce platelets.

Antibodies

specialized proteins of the immune system that help fight infections. They can also be created to recognize proteins on cancer cells, as in some types of lymphoma treatments.

spleen tends to remove platelets coated with antibody from the blood circulation. Signs of a low platelet count include bleeding that occurs spontaneously or with only minimal trauma, such as nose bleeding or menstrual periods that are heavier than normal. When a low platelet count results in an increased risk of bleeding, platelet transfusions may be required to lower this risk.

The platelet count can sometimes be high in patients with lymphoma or other cancers because the body may react to the presence of cancer, infection, or some types of inflammation by making more platelets. The platelet count will generally return to normal with treatment.

9. How does the immune system fight infection?

The immune system uses two main strategies for attacking foreign proteins. The first uses the **humoral immune response**, and the foot soldiers for this mode of attack are the B cells. The other arm of the attack is the **cellular immune response**, which the T cells predominantly perform. The two strategies generally act by cooperating with each other in any attempt to eliminate a foreign substance.

The humoral immune response uses antibodies to eliminate foreign protein. Antibodies are Y-shaped proteins that can attach to the foreign protein in much the same way as a key fits in a lock. The arms of the Y bind to the foreign protein, and the leg attaches to another type of immune cell called a **phagocyte**, which then removes the foreign protein coated with antibody from the circulation.

Humoral immune response

an immune response that uses antibodies rather than cells to destroy an antigen (foreign protein).

Cellular immune response

the part of the immune response that uses lymphocytes to directly remove antigens.

Phagocyte

a cell that scavenges other cells.

When specific B cells recognize a substance as foreign, they turn into cells that can secrete antibodies. These cells are called **plasma cells,** which are found mostly in the spleen but are common in the bone marrow. Normally, there is one pool of B cells for each different foreign protein that anybody might encounter over the course of a lifetime. When exposed to that foreign protein, the specific pool of B cells that can react to that foreign protein is stimulated to develop into plasma cells. The resulting population of plasma cells produces a specific antibody that is capable of attaching itself to the foreign protein. The attachment of the antibody to the foreign protein marks that protein for removal from circulation and the body's subsequent destruction.

Plasma cells

the most mature type of B cell, they produce immunoglobulins and are the malignant cell in multiple myeloma.

Some of the B cells that recognize a foreign substance do not become plasma cells but instead act to recruit T cells to help fight the foreign invader. The type of immune response that results from T-cell involvement is called the cellular immune response, which does not use antibodies; instead, T cells, when activated by an encounter with the foreign protein, create chemicals called **lymphokines** that in turn activate an entire host of immune cells, including phagocytes, with the end result of eliminating the infection. Lymphokines and similar substances called **cytokines** are responsible for many of the symptoms, such as fever and aching, that occur during viral infections such as the flu.

Lymphokines

chemicals that are produced by lymphocytes and help in coordinating the immune response.

Cytokines

chemicals produced by T-lymphoctyes to generate an immune response.

10. How is the immune system important in lymphoma?

The immune system is designed to recognize foreign proteins, and the way it does this is most evident in the responses seen with infection; however, the immune system also plays a role in surveying the body for

The Basics

abnormal cells that, if not removed, can become cancers. All cancers start out as an abnormality that occurs in a single cell. This abnormal cell develops a feature that somehow allows it to survive better than its normal counterparts—that is, it develops a survival advantage. In order to recognize an abnormal cell as foreign, the cells of the immune system need to recognize a protein on the surface of the cell as abnormal. In lymphoma and many other cancers, the proteins on the surface of the lymphoma cell appear normal, explaining why the immune response against the cancer is so weak.

All lympho-mas arise from abnormalities in cells of the immune system.

All lymphomas arise from abnormalities in cells of the immune system, specifically the lymphocytes. In some cases, the lymphoma may occur as a result of some lymphocytes overreacting to certain types of infections. It is widely thought that many tissues develop small numbers of abnormal cells that have the potential to develop into cancers, but the immune system's recognition of these cells results in their safe removal. Therefore, a failure of the immune system to recognize the abnormal cells before they become a cancer is one mechanism whereby cancers, including lymphoma, can occur.

Currently, an interesting and promising area of research is focusing on ways to make cancer cells more recognizable to the immune system. Cancer vaccines are designed with this goal in mind, and ongoing clinical trials are demonstrating interesting results in some types of lymphoma. One approach to treating lymphoma involves tricking the body into recognizing the lymphoma cells as foreign by using the abnormal lymphocytes as a vaccine.

In some types of lymphoma, characterized by slow growth and often not treated for periods of time, the lymph node enlargement can wax and wane. This may reflect the immune system's attempt to control the lymphoma. This observation suggests that ways to enhance the immune system may allow for improved control of these types of lymphoma.

The treatment of lymphoma itself can have a significant impact on the immune system. The presence of lymphoma can impair the ability of the immune system to respond to infection, and this can be improved with treatment by controlling the lymphoma; however, the treatment of the lymphoma itself can further impair the functioning of the immune system.

The Basics

PART TWO

Diagnosis and Classification of Lymphoma

What is lymphoma?

What is Hodgkin's disease?

More . . .

11. What is lymphoma?

Lymphoma

cancer of the lymphocytes.

Lymphoma is cancer of the lymphatic system, particularly the lymphocytes, in which an abnormality occurs in one lymphocyte that allows the cell to divide and grow abnormally. Like all cancer cells, the abnormal lymphocyte does not obey the signals that control normal cell behavior. This allows more of the abnormal cells to grow, eventually developing into a large collection of the abnormal lymphocytes, which when big enough for an examination or an x-ray to detect is called a tumor or mass. A **biopsy** can then be done that allows the lymphoma to be diagnosed.

Biopsy

the removal of tissue or a fluid sample for microscopic examination.

Most commonly, the abnormal growth of lymphocytes occurs in the lymph nodes, which then become enlarged. Abnormal lymphocytes can also collect in the bone marrow, the blood, the spleen, or other sites such as the gut, lungs, or brain. It is not uncommon for the skin to be involved.

Lymphoma is actually a term that applies to many different disorders.

Lymphoma is actually a term that applies to many different disorders that all have many features in common (the features described here).

Pathologist

a physician who makes the diagnosis of lymphoma and other cancers from evaluating biopsies and other surgical specimens under the microscope.

The two main types of lymphoma are Hodgkin's disease and non-Hodgkin's lymphoma. Hodgkin's disease is named after Thomas Hodgkin, an English **pathologist** who originally described the disease in the 1800s. The specific type of lymphoma, Hodgkin's or non-Hodgkin's, depends on the nature of the abnormal lymphocytes and how they look to the pathologist when he or she examines them under the microscope.

12. What is Hodgkin's disease?

Hodgkin's disease, also called Hodgkin's lymphoma, is a cancer of the lymphatic system that most commonly affects people in their late teens or early 20s or people in their 50s. It is unclear why this cancer affects people more at these ages. Four main types of Hodgkin's disease exist (Table 1), and a lymph node biopsy, seen under a microscope, will provide the correct diagnosis.

13. What is non-Hodgkin's lymphoma?

Non-Hodgkin's lymphoma, or NHL, is actually a term applied to many different types of lymphatic cancer, including all types that are apart from Hodgkin's disease. After the surgeon removes the lymph node, the pathologist can generally tell your doctor the exact type of the lymphoma by examining the lymph node and the individual cells under the microscope. They also do more specialized studies to identify the exact type of the individual cells that make up the tumor. The type of NHL you have will help determine your treatment. There are too many types to discuss in one short question, so most of the different varieties of NHL are described individually in Part 3.

Because there are so many different types of non-Hodgkin's lymphoma, it is important to have a good

The type of NHL you have will help determine your treatment.

Table 1   The different types of Hodgkin's disease

Type	Prevalence
Nodular Sclerosing	Most common (75%)
Lymphocyte Predominant	
Mixed Cellularity	
Lymphocyte Depleted	Least common (less than 5%)

classification system that will group those lymphomas that behave in a similar fashion or that require a similar type of treatment. This system allows your doctor to predict how the lymphoma is likely to respond to treatment, to decide on the correct treatment, and to determine **prognosis**. The system of classification is discussed further in Question 18.

Prognosis

a prediction of the course that a disease will take.

14. What are the symptoms of lymphoma?

The most common findings of lymphoma are enlarged or swollen lymph nodes (called **lymphadenopathy**), which most commonly occur in your neck, armpit, or groin (Table 2).

Lymphadenopathy

enlarged lymph nodes.

Occasionally, groin lymph node enlargement can result in swelling of the leg on the same side. Although lymphoma-enlarged lymph nodes are usually painless, some pain may occur, especially if the nodes are growing very fast. As the lymphatic system branches all throughout the body, these swellings may occur anywhere, even in places where you or your doctor cannot feel them easily. If the lymph node swelling develops in your stomach area or intestinal tract, you may have abdominal pain and/or bloating or a feeling of getting full faster than normal. When the lymph nodes in the chest become involved, cough, shortness of breath, or

Table 2   The symptoms of lymphoma

Lymphoma symptoms are not specific. Not all people with lymphoma will experience all symptoms, and some will have symptoms not listed here. Common symptoms include:

- Fatigue
- Painless swelling of lymph glands (rarely painful)
- Fevers
- Night sweats
- Weight loss

chest pain may develop. Sometimes, if the lymph nodes in the center of the chest get big very fast, they can cause **superior vena cava syndrome**, which is pressure that the lymph nodes put on veins, resulting in slowing of the blood flow returning from your arms and head back to your heart. This can result in headache, swelling (possibly affecting the head, neck, and arms), difficulty breathing, or vision problems.

If bone marrow is involved, you may experience anemia that results in generalized weakness and **fatigue**. Bleeding may result from a low platelet count, or infections may occur as a result of a low white blood cell count. Occasionally, lymphoma can also involve the brain or spinal cord, resulting in headaches, double vision, or weakness in an arm or leg. With involvement of the spinal cord, back pain, leg weakness, numbness, or problems related to the control of bowel or bladder function may occur. Most commonly, the spinal cord itself is not involved, but the lymphoma may press on the spinal cord, resulting in these problems. If any symptoms of spinal cord involvement occur, you should see your doctor immediately or, if at night, go to the emergency room, as any delay could result in paralysis.

Other symptoms that can occur, regardless of the site of the lymphoma, may include fever, night sweats, and weight loss (these are the **B symptoms** that are mentioned in Question 19); when these symptoms are present to a significant degree, they indicate a more aggressive lymphoma.

Many people with lymphoma won't have any symptoms. In these cases, the enlarged lymph nodes may be

Superior vena cava syndrome

a condition where the blood flow back to the heart is decreased due to obstruction, usually by very big lymph nodes.

Fatigue

tiredness, particularly the debilitating, continuous tiredness that signals illness or disease.

B symptoms

fevers, night sweats, and weight loss that may occur individually or together in lymphoma patients.

Many people with lymphoma won't have any symptoms.

felt in the shower or while lying in bed. Occasionally, your physician may detect them during a routine physical examination; this is more common with the **indolent** lymphomas.

Indolent

usually slow growing.

Another important point to remember is that no symptoms are unique to lymphoma. Most of the time symptoms from something other than lymphoma will be seen. In most people with enlarged, painful lymph nodes, various infections are a much more common cause; but if the lymph node remains large or continues to grow, especially if it is not painful, you should see your physician who will consider a biopsy.

15. How is lymphoma diagnosed?

The diagnosis of lymphoma is made from a lymph node biopsy, which involves obtaining a sample of an enlarged lymph node and examining it under a microscope. Before the biopsy, which a surgeon usually performs, your primary care doctor will have carried out a careful medical history, a physical examination, and some blood tests.

The biopsy is done in the doctor's office or the hospital and, depending on which part of the body is involved, can be done with either a local or general anesthetic. Sometimes a needle alone is used to obtain a small sample of cells in a procedure called a **fine needle aspiration** (FNA). This is easier to do than a biopsy. However, for the purposes of diagnosing the lymphoma, it is generally not quite as good as taking out the entire lymph node. When examining the cells under a microscope, it is important to see an overview of the pattern of how the cells appear (the bird's eye view) rather than just looking at the individual cells. This feature of the

Fine needle aspiration

a procedure to obtain a sample of tissue using a small needle.

biopsy, termed the **lymph node architecture**, is an important part of a lymphoma diagnosis. Nevertheless, there are times when it is very hard to remove an entire lymph node, or too many risks are involved in using a general anesthetic; thus, a fine needle aspirate may be adequate to make the diagnosis.

After removal, the lymph node is sent to the laboratory where the lymph node tissue is treated with special chemicals to "fix" it, which results in preservation of the tissue. Then it is cut into very thin sections, placed on glass slides, and stained, making it ready for the pathologist to examine. The staining allows the different cells and structures within the lymph node to be distinguished from each other.

The pathologist examines the lymph node to see first whether the cells are normal or abnormal. It is common for lymph nodes to become enlarged in reaction to infection or inflammation. Next, he or she sees whether the abnormality is **benign** or **malignant**. If it is benign, it is not harmful and not cancerous. If it is malignant, it can either be lymphoma or a different type of cancer that has spread to the lymph node.

After the pathologist has decided that it is lymphoma, distinguishing between Hodgkin's disease and non-Hodgkin's lymphoma becomes important. The types of cells and their pattern under the microscope are the most helpful for this purpose.

Another helpful test, called **flow cytometry**, provides a way of examining and identifying different types of cells by seeing particular proteins that exist on their surface. Different lymphomas have particular patterns

Lymph node architecture
the structure of lymph nodes when they are seen under a microscope.

Benign
a growth that is not cancerous.

Malignant
cancerous.

Flow cytometry
a procedure for examining the proteins present on the surface of cells.

of protein expression that help to determine the exact type of lymphoma. Flow cytometry will be performed in almost all cases in which lymphoma is suspected.

As you will see, given that there are so many different types of lymphoma and the differences between many of them can be very subtle, it can sometimes be very difficult to be sure of the type of lymphoma that you have. In these rare cases, it is a good idea to get a second opinion from another pathologist. This is especially true if knowing the exact type will change the way the lymphoma will be treated. In many cases, the difference is so subtle that it will not affect the treatment, and from a practical point of view, the distinction is less important.

16. Could my lymphoma have been diagnosed earlier, and does it make a difference?

When a lump is discovered, the internist or family doctor will usually want to keep an eye on the lump, as most lumps are due to benign causes and go away without treatment. In the vast majority of cases, the doctor is right to suspect an infection and to prescribe antibiotics, thus sparing many patients from the process of an unnecessary biopsy.

However, if you find out that you have a lymphoma instead of an infection, it is natural to wonder why the diagnosis was not made sooner. It might be good to remember that when your lymphoma was first diagnosed, you may have been feeling great and just happened to notice a lump, although some nonspecific symptoms may have also been present. Most doctors will have no hesitation in discussing your concerns about the timing of the diagnosis; if this is not done, your questions may linger and distract you from coping with everything else that is happening.

The question of whether diagnosing the lymphoma earlier makes a difference can be complicated. Lymphoma is very different from other cancers (such as breast, bowel, or lung cancer) in this respect. In these and other cancers, the ability to cure the disease largely depends on whether the cancer has spread from the site where it initially started. This is not true for lymphoma because the lymphatic system where the cancer begins is distributed throughout the body. Spreading from one place to another does not have the same worrisome implications as it does in these other cancers. The ability to cure lymphoma depends more on what particular type of lymphoma you have—whether it is indolent or aggressive rather than whether it is in only one spot. That is not to say that having a lymphoma confined to one or two areas is not a better situation than having a lymphoma that has spread; nevertheless, lymphoma that has spread can also be cured.

Lymphoma that has spread can also be cured.

17. What causes lymphoma?

The cause of lymphoma in most people remains unknown; it is easier, in fact, to list what does *not* cause lymphoma. No association has been made with smoking or alcohol use. Particular diets or lifestyles in general do not appear to increase the chance of developing lymphoma. Lymphoma does not occur as a result of previous injury, and it is not related to being overweight. Lymphoma cannot spread from one person to another.

Many scientists have tried to identify certain things that could cause lymphoma. In most cases, the evidence for an association is weak, although exposure to certain chemicals such as insecticides or pesticides over prolonged periods of time may result in a higher incidence of lymphoma. These chemicals have been implicated in a higher incidence of non-Hodgkin's lymphoma among farm workers in some rural areas of the United States.

An abnormal immune system increases the chances of developing lymphoma.

It is very clear that an abnormal immune system increases the chances of developing lymphoma. The most dramatic example of this is **acquired immunodeficiency syndrome** (AIDS), caused by the **human immunodeficiency virus** (HIV). This virus infects lymphocytes, resulting in a markedly abnormal immune system, which is followed by the development of lymphoma in some patients. Abnormal immune systems can also be acquired after heart, lung, kidney, or liver transplants, for which recipients are kept on drugs to prevent rejection, usually for the rest of their lives. These drugs inhibit the normal function of the lymphocytes, as it is these cells that can cause rejection. Lymphoma occurs more commonly in these people.

Acquired immunodeficiency syndrome (AIDS)

the syndrome resulting from infection with the human immunodeficiency virus (HIV).

Human immunodeficiency virus (HIV)

a virus that attacks the human immune system, leaving the carrier prone to infections.

Epstein Barr virus

the virus that causes infectious mononucleosis and can cause lymphocytes to grow abnormally.

Another virus that may cause lymphoma is the **Epstein-Barr virus**, which infects many people without causing illness and is the cause of infectious mononucleosis (popularly know as "glandular fever" or "mono" and often called "the kissing disease," as it is common among adolescents and is spread through saliva). In the laboratory, this virus can make B lymphocytes grow abnormally. Some lymphoma patients have Epstein-Barr virus present in their lymphoma cells, suggesting that the virus may be involved in the development of their lymphoma; however, another explanation is that the immune abnormality that allowed the lymphoma to develop also allowed the Epstein-Barr virus infection to occur. This would make Epstein-Barr virus an innocent bystander infection rather than the cause of the lymphoma. Currently, the treatment of lymphoma is usually not different when Epstein-Barr virus is or is not present. Therefore, testing is not done on a routine basis. An exception to this is when lymphoma occurs after transplant when testing for Epstein-Barr virus may be important.

An unusual type of lymphoma occurs in some people infected with the **human T-cell lymphotropic virus type 1 (HTLV–1)**. This virus occurs most frequently in Japan and parts of the Caribbean and can result in a form of T-cell lymphoma that can be very aggressive but fortunately is quite rare. Recently, it has also been suggested that the **hepatitis C virus (HCV)** may increase the chances of developing lymphoma. This is worrisome, as the number of people infected with this virus has increased dramatically over the past 20 years.

18. How is lymphoma classified?

Your doctor will use **lymphoma classification** to decide what treatment is necessary for your type of lymphoma. Lymphoma classification groups the many different types of non-Hodgkin's lymphoma into a more manageable number of categories. The different lymphomas are categorized according to similar characteristics that can predict the prognosis and determine the best type of treatment. A good classification is also necessary to carry out the **clinical trials** that are vital for improving the treatment of lymphoma. Generally, these trials compare groups of patients receiving different treatments to decide which treatment is better. The classification allows the researcher to determine that similar types of patients were treated in each group. Any difference in the outcome is then more

Human T-cell lymphotropic virus type 1

a virus that can cause leukemia by infecting T lymphocytes.

Hepatitis C virus

one of the viruses that can infect the liver and cause chronic liver inflammation.

Lymphoma classification

a system to organize the many different types of lymphoma.

Clinical trials

research studies evaluating promising new treatments in patients.

likely due to the treatment rather than to differences in the groups of patients treated. Hodgkin's disease is classified as shown earlier in Table 1. The classification of non-Hodgkin's lymphoma, on the other hand, is much more complicated and has changed many times as we learn more about the biology and behavior of the different types of lymphoma. The classification is very useful in helping your doctor give you an idea about how the lymphoma is likely to behave—whether it will be slow growing and can be managed, possibly for many years, or whether it requires intense chemotherapy in an attempt to cure the lymphoma. A useful classification for both you and your doctor is the **Working Formulation** system, which determines whether your type of lymphoma is low, intermediate, or high grade. (The newer classifications use the term "indolent" for the low-grade lymphomas and the term "aggressive" for the intermediate- and high-grade lymphomas. You will see both terms used during your reading.) The distinction between these types is important for choosing the right treatment. Each of these categories includes a number of different lymphomas that generally behave in a similar fashion and are treated in similar ways. The pathologist makes the distinction between the different categories when he or she examines the lymph node biopsy under the microscope. The features of the individual lymphocytes and the way that they are arranged in the lymph node allow the pathologist to determine whether your lymphoma is low, intermediate, or high grade.

As a classification system gets put into practice and is used for large numbers of patients, it becomes apparent that there are cases of lymphoma that do not fall neatly into any one category. This is a problem if there are

Working Formulation

one of the lymphoma classifications.

enough of these cases. As scientific advances have allowed a much better understanding of what is happening in individual cancer cells at the molecular level, our ability to distinguish between the different lymphomas has increased. This has led to a newer classification of the lymphomas, called the Revised European American Lymphoma classification (REAL classification), which attempts to use all of the currently available information about the lymphoma, including molecular and genetic abnormalities in addition to its appearance under the microscope. The World Health Organization has further revised this classification. From a practical point of view, however, the Working Formulation remains very useful, and therefore, we discuss lymphomas using this system throughout the text.

19. What is meant by the stage of lymphoma?

The **stage** of your lymphoma is I, II, III, or IV. In addition, it is divided into A or B depending on whether B symptoms, including fever, night sweats, and weight loss, have been present (see Question 14 for more on symptoms). A group of lymphoma experts (meeting in Ann Arbor, MI, in 1971) devised the staging system for Hodgkin's disease that is thus known as the **Ann Arbor Staging System**. Since then, it has been applied very successfully to non-Hodgkin's lymphoma and remains the best staging system available for both Hodgkin's disease and non-Hodgkin's lymphoma.

Staging is very important information for every patient with lymphoma, as it provides a common language for doctors and patients to describe how much lymphoma

Stage

a reference to the number of places in the body affected by lymphoma or other cancer.

Ann Arbor Staging System

Used to describe the areas in the body affected by the lymphoma. It was created at a conference held in Ann Arbor, Michigan.

is present and where it is distributed throughout the body. It is used for all lymphomas, regardless of whether they are indolent or aggressive. It is vital information for deciding on the correct treatment and can also help in estimating the prognosis.

There are four stages described in the Ann Arbor system (the staging system uses Roman numerals). It divides lymphoma into limited stage for stage I and II and more extensive stage for stage III and IV.

Stage I refers to involvement of a single lymph node region. Stage II refers to two or more lymph node regions on the same side of the diaphragm (the large muscle that separates the chest from the abdomen and is important for breathing). Stage III is where lymph node regions on both sides of the diaphragm are involved (for the purposes of staging, the spleen is included as a lymph node region). Stage IV includes involvement of disease in lymph node regions and also non-lymph node sites such as the bone marrow, liver, lungs, gut, or skin (Table 3).

Table 3   Staging of lymphoma*

Stage 1	One lymph node area involved
Stage 2	Two or more lymph node areas on the *same side* of the diaphragm
Stage 3	Lymph nodes involved on *both sides* of the diaphragm
Stage 4	Any of the above with involvement of sites other than lymph nodes (most commonly the bone marrow, liver or lungs)
B symptoms	Fever, night sweats, or significant weight loss

*After designation of the stage based on the sites of involvement, patients are categorized as either A (if no B symptoms are present) or B (if B symptoms are present).

The presence of lymphoma involving a site other than the lymph nodes or spleen generally implies stage IV unless the involvement is directly from a lymph node. For example, if there is involvement of the lung directly next to involved lymph nodes in the chest, the subscript E is written beside the stage. Thus, III_E would indicate that lymph nodes on both sides of the diaphragm are involved and that lymphoma has extended out from a lymph node into a surrounding organ. Stage IV refers to lymphoma involving a non-lymphoid organ such as the bone marrow, liver, or lung where it is not directly spreading from a lymph node.

As mentioned, the stage is further characterized as A or B. If B symptoms exist, then it is stage B; otherwise, it is stage A. In general, stage B suggests that the lymphoma is more aggressive.

20. How is staging performed?

Until about 10 years ago, many people with lymphoma underwent a surgical procedure called **laparotomy** for staging. This procedure involved opening the abdomen, taking samples or biopsies of many lymph nodes, performing a liver biopsy, and removing the spleen. The spleen, lymph node, and liver biopsies would then be examined under a microscope to determine lymphoma involvement. This surgical staging procedure was performed mostly in patients with limited-stage Hodgkin's disease but also in some patients with non-Hodgkin's lymphoma.

The laparotomy was necessary because **computed tomography** (CT) scans done to look for lymphoma in the liver or spleen can be normal unless these organs are enlarged. A normal-sized liver or spleen may still be involved with lymphoma and may appear entirely

Laparotomy
surgery involving an incision to look directly into the abdomen.

Computed tomography (CT scan)
a specialized type of x-ray that creates a detailed cross-sectional view of the body.

normal on a scan. In such cases, the only way to tell was to do a surgical biopsy; however, because this was major surgery, it was only performed if absolutely necessary for treatment planning to know whether the lymphoma was limited (stage I or stage II) or more extensive (stage III or stage IV). Because of differences in the way Hodgkin's disease and non-Hodgkin's lymphoma behave and are treated, this was not as important in non-Hodgkin's lymphoma. Nowadays, with improved imaging methods and treatment and other ways to predict involvement in the liver and spleen, this surgery is rarely performed.

Staging now relies on a physical examination, x-rays, CT scans, and bone marrow examination. **Positron emission tomography** (PET) scanning is also useful in some situations (Table 4).

Positron emission tomography (PET)
radiologic studies that use the abnormal sugar metabolism of cancer cells to identify metastatic deposits..

The physical examination for staging focuses on determining whether there is enlargement of the lymph nodes, liver, and spleen. On examination, enlarged lymph nodes in the head and neck region, the armpit (axilla), and also the groin can be detected. Lymph

Table 4   Tests for staging of lymphoma

Tests necessary for staging	Tests sometimes required
Physical examination	CT scan of neck and chest
Chest x-ray	PET scan
CT scan of abdomen and pelvis	Bone marrow biopsy on both sides
Bone marrow biopsy	Gallium scan
	Spinal tap

nodes are occasionally felt in the elbow or knee region. In order for the spleen to be felt, it needs to be two to three times larger than normal. Radiologic studies (x-ray, CT, or **magnetic resonance imaging** [MRI]) are needed to see the lymph nodes that your doctor cannot feel. These include the lymph nodes between the lungs (known as the **mediastinal nodes**) and the lymph nodes in the abdomen (known as the **retroperitoneal lymph nodes** and **mesenteric lymph nodes**). In people without lymphoma, lymph nodes are normally present at these sites but are not enlarged, measuring up to only 1 cm.

The most commonly used radiologic test for staging is the CT scan (also known as a CAT scan). The x-ray camera takes many individual pictures at different angles, and these are then combined into multiple, computer-generated, cross-sectional images at each level that need to be examined. Often, scans are obtained of the chest, abdomen, and pelvis. Many physicians will obtain a CT scan of the abdomen and pelvis only and will use a plain x-ray of the chest to evaluate the lymph nodes above the diaphragm. The plain x-ray of the chest often gives as much information for staging as the CT scan. A CT scan of the neck can be obtained if there is doubt about involvement of the neck lymph nodes. MRI scans can also be used for staging and may be useful instead of a CT scan under special circumstances. In order to get the best CT scan pictures, **contrast dye** is given orally and intravenously. The dye allows better visualization between the lymph nodes and other tissues, including blood vessels and gut; however, the dye can occasionally affect kidney function. If your doctor feels that you are at risk for this side effect, an MRI can be used instead of a CT

Magnetic resonance imaging

a technique based on the use of magnetic fields to produce images of body parts.

Mediastinal nodes

lymph nodes present in the area between the lungs.

Retroperitoneal lymph nodes

the most common lymph nodes present in the abdomen.

Mesenteric lymph nodes

the lymph nodes present in the abdomen in the tissue that anchors the bowel.

Contrast dye

a chemical that is injected for certain x-rays including CT scans and MRI scans that results in better contrast pictures.

scan. The contrast dye can also cause allergic reactions that require premedication with a small dose of steroids before the CT scan. CT and MRI scans are very good for examining the size of lymph nodes but do not tell you definitively whether big lymph nodes contain lymphoma. At the time of diagnosis, if a lymph node biopsy confirms lymphoma, it is reasonable to assume that other big lymph nodes are also involved with lymphoma; however, after treatment, lymph nodes can remain enlarged due to large amounts of inflammation or scar tissue. These nodes will still look big on a CT or MRI scan. It is important in this situation to be able to tell the difference between big lymph nodes that lymphoma causes versus big nodes that scar tissue causes. Another biopsy is the only way to be absolutely sure; however, a newer test called a PET scan may be very helpful. The PET scan involves injection of a radioactive tracer into the bloodstream. Active lymphoma cells pick up the tracer, and, therefore, even if the lymph nodes are not enlarged, areas of lymphoma can still be detected with a positron camera. A PET scan can also be useful for staging lymphoma when it is first diagnosed.

Lymphangiogram

an x-ray study of lymph glands after they are injected with a dye.

Although a **lymphangiogram** is an older test that is rarely done nowadays, as it is technically a difficult test for the radiologist to perform, it has been used for staging. Because it is rarely done, few radiologists have much experience in either performing or interpreting the test. The procedure involves injecting dye into the lymph vessels of both feet. These vessels are very tiny and difficult to find. Once injected, the dye travels to the lymph nodes in the groin and abdomen and can show abnormal lymph nodes even if they are not larger than normal. The test has been most useful for the accurate staging of Hodgkin's disease, but newer tests provide similar information.

A **gallium scan,** another test that can be used for staging, involves giving a small amount of radioactive gallium as an intravenous injection. After the injection, scanning is performed 2 and 3 days later. Some lymphomas take up the gallium, whereas others do not. In order to know whether a gallium scan will be useful, a baseline scan needs to be obtained before treatment. This scan tells you whether your lymphoma takes up gallium; if so, additional gallium scans will be useful to follow the response to treatment. It has been most useful in Hodgkin's disease but may also be useful for non-Hodgkin's lymphoma. Similar to the PET scan, the gallium scan can be useful to evaluate enlarged lymph nodes that persist after treatment, helping to differentiate between scar tissue and active lymphoma.

Gallium scan

a nuclear medicine test that uses gallium to show areas of lymphoma within the body.

A bone marrow examination is also part of the staging evaluation. Occasionally, it is important to do this test on both sides of the hipbone (a bilateral biopsy).

21. How is a bone marrow examination performed?

Lymphoma often involves the bone marrow. When this occurs, production of all the normal blood cells may be decreased, resulting in a low red cell count (anemia), a low platelet count (**thrombocytopenia**), or a low white cell count (**leukopenia**). Most patients who are being evaluated for lymphoma require a bone marrow examination. When staging lymphoma for the first time, a bone marrow sample may be obtained from both sides of the hip because only one side may contain the lym-

Thrombocytopenia

a low platelet count.

Leukopenia

a low white blood cell count.

phoma. Bone marrow sampling is important as it affects the choice of treatment and is also frequently necessary for evaluating the response to treatment.

The bone marrow is obtained from the hipbone at the back, generally at the site of the "dimples of Venus," next to the tailbone. This procedure, usually done in 20 to 30 minutes in the outpatient clinic, can be done with the patient lying either on his or her side or front. The bone marrow test has two parts: bone marrow aspiration, which refers to the sampling of the liquid part of the bone marrow within the marrow cavity, and bone marrow biopsy, which involves taking a tiny core of the bone that when looked at under the microscope shows the bird's eye view of the marrow within the bone.

First, the skin over the site on the hipbone is cleansed with a disinfectant and then numbed with local anesthetic, usually lidocaine. Next, the area down to the surface of the bone is numbed. The surface of the bone can be particularly sensitive when the lidocaine is first injected, as the lidocaine causes a stinging sensation. Next, a very small incision is made. The bone marrow needle is then drilled into the marrow cavity with a gentle corkscrew type of motion. A pressure sensation usually accompanies this. The inside of the bone marrow is liquid, and a small amount (2 to 5 cc) is then sucked out with the needle. This only takes a couple of seconds, but for many people it is the worst part of the procedure. The bone marrow itself cannot be anesthetized, and when sucked out can feel like a very strange pulling sensation in the hip and also down the leg. The person doing the procedure can help by talking to you, describing each step, and giving you a warning before the marrow is withdrawn. This discomfort should only last a couple of seconds.

The second part of the test involves doing the biopsy. The biopsy needle is placed in the same area on the hipbone, and a hollow needle is drilled into the bone. Again, this should feel only like a pressure sensation. The needle is then removed with the piece of bone inside. Pressure is held over the site to prevent bleeding, and a bandage is applied to the area. This is the end of the procedure.

22. How do I prepare for a bone marrow test?

For many people, the worst part of the test is waiting for the appointment. The build-up of anxiety may actually increase the pain and discomfort associated with the test. Thus, a shorter appointment time may be helpful. If you are taking aspirin or a similar type of drug that prevents platelets from working properly, ask your doctor whether it should be stopped. Many patients find it helpful to have a friend or relative accompany them to the appointment. Usually a sedative is not necessary for the procedure, so patients can drive themselves to and from the appointment if necessary. In fact, many patients return to work after the test.

The worst part of the bone marrow test is waiting for the appointment.

After the test, you can be up and about as normal. You may feel some aching discomfort in the area of the biopsy after the local anesthetic wears off, but this should only last for 1 or 2 days. A mild painkiller such as Tylenol is usually effective in controlling the discomfort. Aspirin or similar medications are to be avoided, as they can increase the chance of bleeding. Bleeding from the site of the biopsy can occur, and simply applying pressure will generally stop most bleeding. It is very rare for an infection or serious bleeding to result from a bone marrow test.

PART THREE

Types of Lymphoma

What type of lymphoma do I have?

What is low-grade lymphoma?

What is intermediate-grade lymphoma?

More . . .

23. What type of lymphoma do I have?

The type of lymphoma that you have depends on how the lymphoma biopsy looked under the microscope; moreover (as discussed in Question 14), non-Hodgkin's lymphoma can be separated into three broad categories that give you and your doctor a good indication of how your particular lymphoma may respond to treatment. Each of the three categories— low (indolent), intermediate, or high grade (aggressive)—behaves differently and requires a different approach to treatment. Each of the categories also includes a number of different lymphomas (discussed in the Questions 24–42).

NON-HODGKIN'S LYMPHOMA

24. What is low-grade lymphoma?

Indolent lymphomas generally are slow-growing, and their appearance under the microscope provides the diagnosis. The lymphocytes that make up the tumors are generally small and tend to grow in circular groups of cells called **nodules** or **follicles**. This is similar to how lymphocytes appear in normal lymph nodes. This pattern of tumor growth is not always the case in indolent lymphoma, however, because the lymphocytes can appear distributed evenly throughout the lymph node, taking on a diffuse appearance. Because the distinction of the different lymphomas using just the appearance under the microscope is not always reliable, other special tests are done to confirm the exact type.

There are several different types of indolent lymphoma, with the most common being the **follicular lymphomas**, of which there are three subtypes: Type 1 consists of mostly small-cleaved cells, whereas types 2

Follicles

round structures containing lymphocytes; also called nodules.

Follicular lymphomas

lymphomas composed of lymphocytes organized into round structures.

and 3 each have increasing numbers of larger cells mixed in with the smaller cells. The presence of the larger cells may indicate a more aggressive type of indolent lymphoma. Another type of low-grade lymphoma is small lymphocytic lymphoma (SLL), which does not have the circular or nodular pattern of lymphocyte growth when examined under the microscope. This lymphoma is very closely related to chronic lymphocytic leukemia (CLL), in which similar types of lymphocytes are found in the lymph nodes and bone marrow in addition to the blood. In lymphoma, the abnormal lymphocytes may also be found in the bloodstream, but the numbers are lower than in CLL. A less common type of indolent lymphoma is marginal zone lymphoma, also called monocytoid B-cell lymphoma or mucosa-associated lymphoid tissue (MALT) lymphoma. These lymphomas tend to grow very slowly and quite commonly involve only one or two sites. Interestingly, when it occurs in the stomach, MALT lymphoma is often associated with a bacteria called *Helicobacter pylori*, which is a prime contributor to other gastric diseases such as ulcers. Giving antibiotics to kill these bacteria can shrink the lymphoma. This type of lymphoma also occurs more commonly in people with autoimmune disease (diseases in which the body forms antibodies against parts of itself, such as rheumatoid arthritis, Sjogren's syndrome, and Hashimoto's thyroiditis).

It is very likely that many patients with indolent lymphoma have had the disease for a long time, possibly years before the diagnosis is made. Usually, when the lymphoma is first diagnosed, it is already present in many different lymph nodes, the spleen, and also usually the bone marrow. This results in a diagnosis of

Many patients with indolent lymphoma have had the disease for a long time, possibly years.

Types of Lymphoma

stage IV lymphoma. Often, a lump or swelling in the neck or groin while taking a shower is the first sign that you will notice. Infection is a much more common cause of lymph node enlargement than lymphoma, and therefore it is common for the doctor to recommend observing the swelling for a few weeks to see whether it will go away on its own. Sometimes antibiotics will be prescribed. In most people, the lymph node swelling does go away. If not, a surgeon may consider performing a lymph node biopsy.

The type of lymphoma determines how it should be treated. Although many different treatments can help to control the lymphoma, none of them have been able to cure the indolent lymphomas. Therefore, the aim of treatment for this type of lymphoma is to allow you to feel as well as possible for as long as possible. Many people with indolent lymphoma will feel perfectly well when the lymphoma is first diagnosed and may not need any treatment at that time.

25. What is intermediate-grade lymphoma?

Intermediate-grade lymphomas grow faster than the indolent lymphomas. They include a number of different types of lymphoma that can be distinguished under the microscope. These lymphomas are often curable, and therefore a patient diagnosed with intermediate-grade lymphoma should receive treatment regardless of whether symptoms are present. The most common of the intermediate-grade lymphomas is **diffuse large B cell lymphoma**. Because these lymphomas are relatively fast growing, they often involve fewer lymph nodes at diagnosis. Although the indo-

Diffuse large B cell lymphoma

the most common type of intermediate grade lymphoma.

lent lymphomas are often stage IV, the intermediate-grade lymphomas are often stage I or stage II. However, lymphoma is frequently present in the bone marrow, resulting in a diagnosis of stage IV lymphoma. It is also not unusual for these lymphomas to involve other areas, including the liver, lung, gut, or even the skin, apart from lymph nodes or bone marrow. If any of these sites are involved in addition to lymph nodes, the lymphoma is stage IV. These lymphomas are more commonly associated with symptoms than the indolent lymphomas.

26. What is high-grade lymphoma?

High-grade lymphomas are the most rapidly growing of the lymphomas and require immediate treatment. They may involve only one or two sites when first diagnosed but are often associated with more prominent symptoms. The best-known lymphoma of this group is **Burkitt's lymphoma**, named for Denis Burkitt, the Irish physician who originally described the disorder. One type, called endemic Burkitt's lymphoma, occurs in children in Africa and often involves the jaw. Another type, the sporadic form, is the most common type of lymphoma that affects children in the United States. A third type of Burkitt's lymphoma occurs in adults, most commonly in people with an abnormal immune system, such as those with AIDS.

Burkitt's lymphoma

a very rapidly growing and aggressive type of lymphoma.

27. What are the different types of indolent lymphoma?

As mentioned in Question 18, the classification of lymphoma has recently changed. Physicians still refer to the terms low, intermediate, and high grade, as these categories provide a useful framework for planning treatment and determining the prognosis. Low-grade and indolent can generally be used interchangeably. The different types of indolent lymphoma are shown in the Table 5.

The three main types of indolent lymphoma are SLL, follicular small cleaved cell lymphoma, and follicular mixed small cleaved and large cell lymphoma. They are included in the low-grade category because they are generally slow growing but cannot usually be cured. Other types of lymphoma such as lymphoplasmacytic lymphoma, which includes Waldenstrom's macroglobulinemia, have also been classified in the indolent lymphoma group.

28. What is SLL?

SLL is very closely related to a type of chronic leukemia called chronic lymphocytic leukemia, or CLL. The "small" in the name refers to the size of the lymphoma cells when seen under the microscope. This

Table 5   Most common types of indolent (low-grade) lymphoma

Small lymphocytic lymphoma (SLL)

Follicular grade 1 and grade 2
    This includes follicular small cleaved cell and follicular small cleaved and large cell lymphoma

Lymphoplasmacytic lymphoma (associated with Waldenstrom's macroglobulinemia)

Marginal zone lymphoma

MALT lymphomas

Splenic lymphoma with villous lymphocytes

is generally a slow-growing lymphoma that occurs mostly in older people. At diagnosis, lymphoma involving the bone marrow is common, and most people are therefore stage IV. The lymphoma can be so similar to CLL that the two diseases are classified together as CLL/SLL in the newest World Health Organization lymphoma classification. The difference between the two diseases really depends on how many of the abnormal cells are present in the blood as compared with the lymph nodes. When the cells are most abundant in the blood, it is called CLL. This type of lymphoma is relatively rare, accounting for less than 5% of all non-Hodgkin's lymphomas. The lymphoma (also CLL) is generally composed of mature B lymphocytes. General management of follicular lymphomas is discussed in Question 29. Similar principles apply to SLL.

29. What are follicular small cleaved cell lymphoma and follicular mixed small cleaved and large cell lymphoma?

These indolent lymphomas are the most common of the non-Hodgkin's lymphomas. The specific type of lymphoma is determined by the number of large cells present among the small lymphocytes (small cleaved cells) that make up the bulk of the lymphoma cells.

More is understood about the abnormalities that occur in the lymphocytes leading to this type of lymphoma than in many other lymphomas. A hallmark of this type of lymphoma is the presence of too much of a protein called Bcl–2. A gene called *bcl–2* produces this protein, and the excess Bcl–2 allows the lymphocyte to live longer than is usual. Because the abnormal lymphocytes fail to die as happens during normal cell turnover, too many lymphocytes accumulate, eventually forming lymph node tumors.

The reason for the overproduction of Bcl–2 is also understood. All humans have 23 pairs of chromosomes—46 in all—that contain many, many genes. The genes are made up of **DNA**, and each contains the fundamental information necessary for the manufacture of a protein. The process responsible for making a protein from the message contained in a gene is normally regulated very closely in order to prevent too much of a protein being produced. Sometimes genes can get moved from one chromosome to another, an event called **translocation**. In the follicular lymphomas, the gene for the production of the Bcl-2 protein (called *bcl-2*) gets moved from chromosome 18 to chromosome 14. On chromosome 14, *bcl-2* is placed next to another gene that gives it instructions to keep producing the Bcl-2 protein. As mentioned previously, the Bcl-2 protein prevents the lymphocyte from dying at the right time. Normal lymphocytes are programmed to die at some point during their normal lifespan. This built-in death program is called **apoptosis** (programmed cell death) and is essentially a cell suicide program. If this process is blocked (e.g., by having too much Bcl-2), lymphocytes accumulate, and lymphoma may result. Many chemotherapy drugs that are useful in lymphoma act by causing lymphocytes to undergo programmed cell death, but when too much Bcl-2 is present the lymphoma can be more resistant to chemotherapy. As a result of this type of research, clinical trials are currently evaluating a compound that can be given to patients to block the Bcl-2 protein from performing its normal function. The hope is that

Translocation

an abnormality of certain chromosomes seen in some cancer cells.

Apoptosis

a process by which normal cells die. Some cancer cells do not die and a failure of cells to undergo apoptosis can contribute to the growth of cancer. It is often referred to as "programmed cell death."

this will then allow cells to die normally and also to respond better to chemotherapy. In October 2002, the Nobel Prize for medicine was awarded to researchers who discovered the basics of this important cell suicide program. The average age at which this type of lymphoma occurs is 55 to 60 years. Males and females are equally affected. Approximately half the patients with stage IV lymphoma will have B symptoms (fevers, night sweats, and weight loss), but the symptoms occur much less frequently in patients with stage I to stage III disease.

Often, the first noticeable symptom is a lump in the neck or groin that may have been present for a while and that is usually painless. It is common for the lymph node swelling to vary in size, maybe even getting smaller (waxing and waning). A biopsy is needed for diagnosis, and it is best if the pathologist removes the entire lymph node (an excisional biopsy) for examination. The pathologist will be more likely to be sure of the diagnosis if more of the node is available. Removing the entire lymph node does not help in treatment, except possibly in the very unlikely event that it is the only site involved (stage I disease). Some doctors may first suggest doing a needle aspiration (putting a needle into the enlarged lymph node and sucking out some cells into a syringe), as this may be sufficient in some cases. The cells are then sent to the pathologist who examines them under the microscope. Unfortunately, because the pathologist is unable to see the "bird's eye" view and sees only the individual cells, it is generally not possible to tell whether there are follicles or nodules (referred to as the architecture of the lymph node), and an excisional biopsy will often be needed in addition.

In some cases, the only enlarged lymph nodes may not be easy to biopsy. Examples include lymph nodes deep inside the chest, between the lungs, or inside the abdomen. In these cases, needle aspirations may be all that are possible. A laparoscopic biopsy (keyhole surgery) can sometimes be performed to obtain a larger piece of the lymph node.

Hematologist/ oncologist

a physician specializing in the treatment of blood disorders and cancer.

You will be referred to a **hematologist/oncologist** after a diagnosis is made. At that point, staging tests are performed, and decisions about treatment are discussed.

30. What is Waldenstrom's macroglobulinemia?

Waldenstrom's macroglobulinemia is a disorder that occurs in patients with a type of indolent lymphoma called lymphoplasmacytic lymphoma. The lymphoma cells occur mostly in the bone marrow and lymph nodes and are generally seen in older individuals, although they occasionally occur in younger people. Waldenstrom's macroglobulinemia refers to a syndrome that is characterized by the presence of too much of an antibody protein called **immunoglobulin M** (IgM), which is normally present in the body and has a role in protecting and fighting against infection. The lymphoma cells, however, produce too much of a single type of IgM, which a special test for **monoclonal antibodies** then detects. The IgM protein produced in Waldenstrom's macroglobulinemia can cause its own problems. The protein circulates in the blood as a very large molecule. Five of these molecules join together to form a very large protein that can cause the blood to become too thick, resulting in a **hyperviscosity** syndrome, which means that the blood is too thick

Immunoglobulin M

one of the 5 different types of antibodies that are part of the immune system.

Monoclonal antibodies

antibodies that bind to a specific target on the surface of lymphoma or other cancer cells.

Hyperviscosity

a condition in which the blood is too thick.

and can result in sluggish blood flow, thus causing symptoms such as dizziness, tiredness, headache, and sometimes bleeding. The serum viscosity test detects hyperviscosity.

Immunoglobulins (such as IgM) are important in preventing infection, and the body produces immunoglobulins as part of the immune response to infection. Part of the immunoglobulin can recognize and attach to bacteria, labeling them for removal from the body. In this same way, IgM may attach to normal body parts such as the lining of nerves or other proteins in the blood. In the case of nerves, this can cause a type of nerve damage called **peripheral neuropathy** (numbness and tingling in the fingers and toes and occasionally weakness). The IgM protein can also cause **Raynaud's syndrome**, a disorder in which the hands get painful and change from white to blue when exposed to the cold. Bleeding problems can also be due to the protein attaching to platelets or other blood proteins that are important for preventing bleeding.

Peripheral neuropathy

a condition caused by damage to the nerves in the arms or legs.

Raynaud's syndrome

a disorder associated with pain and a change in color in the fingers.

The treatment of this type of lymphoma is similar to that of the other types of indolent lymphomas, with the exception that problems related to too much of the IgM might require a different treatment called **plasmapheresis**, which washes the high levels of the abnormal protein from the blood. The lymphoma, like the others in this group, is not curable and is only treated when it is causing problems such as fever or sweats or lowering of normal blood counts. Plasmapheresis can remove the excess IgM, effectively thinning the blood. Sometimes there are no problems related to the lymphoma itself, and thus, treatment with chemotherapy is unnecessary; however, the high

Plasmapheresis

a treatment that consists of removing plasma.

levels of protein may need to be reduced. Plasmapheresis, performed often enough (maybe even once a week) to keep the protein low, may be all that is required. For long-term control, a course of chemotherapy may also be helpful to decrease the protein (IgM) production.

To perform plasmapheresis, two intravenous needles are placed into your arms. One intravenous needle delivers your blood to the plasmapheresis machine. The other returns the blood back to your body. In the machine, which looks much like a kidney dialysis machine, the IgM is separated from the rest of your blood.

31. What is mantle cell lymphoma?

Mantle cell lymphoma

an uncommon type of aggressive lymphoma.

Mantle cell lymphoma has traditionally been included with the indolent lymphomas (because it is generally considered incurable), although most physicians will great it as an aggressive lymphoma; it tends to grow faster, and overall survival may be shorter than with the other types of indolent lymphoma. As a result, most patients will need treatment when the diagnosis is first made.

Mantle cell lymphoma occurs mostly in older adults. Patients often have enlarged lymph nodes at many sites, often with a large liver and spleen because of lymphoma involvement. The bone marrow is also commonly involved. Lymphoma cells may also be found in the bloodstream. Another common site is the gut, especially the colon. Sometimes an abnormality found in the gut at the time of **endoscopy** may lead to the diagnosis of mantle cell lymphoma. If a diagnosis of mantle cell lymphoma has been made, even if there

Endoscopy

a procedure to examine the gut with a fiber-optic light.

are no gastrointestinal symptoms, your physician may want you to undergo endoscopy.

In common with most other types of lymphoma, the cause of mantle cell lymphoma is unknown. As is the case with overproduction of Bcl–2 in the follicular lymphomas, the lymphoma cells in this disorder over-produce a protein called Bcl–1, which causes the abnormal lymphocytes to grow faster and accumulate.

Once the diagnosis is made and staging has been completed, treatment is usually initiated. As with the follicular lymphomas, most patients respond well initially to treatment, sometimes even achieving a complete response (disappearance of all visible evidence of disease); however, on average, the time before the disease comes back is shorter than is the case with the follicular lymphomas.

The treatment of indolent lymphomas, including mantle cell lymphoma, is discussed in Question 52. Some very intensive treatments, including blood stem cell transplantation, may help to improve survival in this type of lymphoma.

32. What are MALT lymphomas?

MALT lymphomas, which stands for mucosa-associated lymphoid tissue and refers to lymphoid tissue that occurs normally in the mucosa (lining) of the gut, **salivary glands**, lung, thyroid, breast, bladder, or kidney, are another uncommon type of indolent lymphoma. The lymphoma is often localized (confined to one area) at the time of diagnosis. Bone marrow involvement is unusual. These lymphomas tend to be slow growing and are more common in people with an

MALT lymphomas
a type of lymphoma that tends to involve lymph glands present in the mucosa (the lining of the gut or other organs).

Salivary glands
the gland that produces saliva.

autoimmune disorder. MALT lymphoma involving the salivary gland occurs more frequently in people with Sjogren's syndrome, and the thyroid lymphoma occurs more frequently in people with Hashimoto's thyroiditis. These are autoimmune disorders in which the body forms antibodies that attack the salivary glands or thyroid gland, respectively.

MALT lymphoma (or MALToma) involving the stomach is often associated with an infection by bacteria called *Helicobacter pylori*. It may be that the presence of the infection causes this specific type of lymphoma to develop or that the bacteria cause ongoing inflammation and irritation to the lining of the stomach. The constant stimulation may cause the abnormal growth of the lymphocytes, ultimately resulting in the development of the lymphoma. Actually, giving antibiotics to patients with both stomach lymphoma and this infection has resulted in remission, even without chemotherapy.

After diagnosis, patients with this type of lymphoma need to undergo staging, as with all other types of lymphoma. If the lymphoma is only present at one site, surgical removal is often recommended, and radiation may also be an option. If the disease is in more than one site, chemotherapy may be recommended.

33. What are marginal zone lymphomas?

Marginal zone lymphomas are closely related to the MALT lymphomas, as they are generally slow growing and tend to occur in older individuals. They have a similar appearance to the MALT lymphomas under the microscope but more frequently occur in the lymph nodes themselves. The name comes from the area in the lymph node surrounding the follicle or nodule that is most abnormal when the lymph node is examined under the microscope. This type of lymphoma can also occur in areas such as the lung or breast without lymphoma being found elsewhere.

34. What is splenic lymphoma with villous lymphocytes?

The MALT lymphomas and marginal zone lymphomas are closely related and differ mostly by where the disease predominates. When the same type of lymphoma exists primarily in the spleen, it is called splenic lymphoma. Sometimes, lymphocytes with characteristic hair-like projections called **villi** can be seen in the blood circulation, resulting in the term "splenic lymphoma with villous lymphocytes." Another term is "splenic marginal zone lymphoma," which is a relatively rare type of indolent lymphoma that is slightly more common in women than men. The diagnosis is sometimes made only after the spleen has been removed. Its features are a large spleen without much lymph node enlargement. Bone marrow involvement is usually present, and abnormal lymphocytes are often seen in the blood. The number of lymphocytes is usually less than that seen in CLL. Like other indolent lymphomas, this disorder is not curable but can usually be controlled for long periods of time. Sometimes the spleen can be removed with no further treatment required for long periods, even many years.

Villi

tiny outcrops of the lining of organs, especially the bowel.

35. Which lymphomas are included in the intermediate-grade category?

These lymphomas include a type of follicular lymphoma that is made up of mostly large cells. The follicular lymphomas that are indolent are composed mostly of small lymphocytes. The most common type of lymphoma in this category is diffuse large B-cell lymphoma, but diffuse small cleaved cell lymphoma and diffuse mixed small and large cell lymphoma are also included.

36. What is diffuse large cell lymphoma?

Diffuse large cell lymphoma is a common type of lymphoma that accounts for approximately 30 to 40% of all lymphomas. It occurs mostly in adults of middle age and older but is not uncommon in younger individuals. The average age at which patients develop this type of lymphoma is 60 years. Many cases are curable with chemotherapy, but if they are not treated, the lymphoma usually grows rapidly and can result in death within a year. Most of these lymphomas arise from B lymphocytes, but 25% arise from T cells. With treatments available today, the outcome, whether of B- or T-cell origin, appears to be similar.

One third of these lymphomas are localized when first diagnosed. The occurrence of the lymphoma at sites other than the lymph nodes, including the gut, lungs, kidneys, and liver, is not uncommon.

Often the first symptom noted may be a rapidly growing lump that is generally painless, but tenderness may be noted because the capsule of the lymph node gets stretched rapidly. Initially, patients may be given antibiotics to treat a suspected infection, as this is a more likely cause of lymph node swelling. If the lymph node does not return to normal over a few weeks with or without antibiotics, a lymph node biopsy should be obtained. Abdominal pain or discomfort, cough, shortness of breath, or a sensation of fullness in the chest or neck may also be the first abnormality noted. Fevers and night sweats may occur, and weight loss may also be noted (these are the B symptoms).

Diffuse large cell lymphoma is actually a "catch-all" phrase for a number of different types of lymphoma. It includes six variants with subtle differences that a pathologist can detect. One of the variants, immuno-blastic lymphoma, is treated the same way as diffuse large cell lymphoma. Other variants include T-cell–rich B-cell lymphoma, lymphomatoid granulomatosis, anaplastic large B cell lymphoma, and plasmablastic lymphoma. These lymphomas all tend to behave simi-larly to diffuse large B-cell lymphoma.

37. What is immunoblastic lymphoma?

Immunoblastic lymphoma has historically been treated as a high-grade lymphoma. Nowadays it is classified along with diffuse large cell lymphoma. Current treatments allow it to be managed similar to diffuse large cell lym-phoma, and many of these lymphomas are curable.

38. What lymphomas are high grade?

This group includes "Burkitt's lymphoma" and "Burkitt's-like" lymphoma. Lymphoblastic lymphoma is also a high-grade lymphoma. Burkitt's and Burkitt's-like lymphomas account for less than 3% of all lymphomas, and only 2% of all lymphomas are lym-phoblastic lymphomas.

39. What is Burkitt's lymphoma?

Burkitt's lymphoma includes very rapidly growing lymphomas but is curable in a high percentage of peo-ple. Both Burkitt's and Burkitt's-like lymphomas behave similarly; however, Burkitt's lymphomas occur predominantly in children whereas Burkitt's-like lymphomas affect older adults.

Burkitt's lymphoma was originally named for Dennis Burkitt, an Irish surgeon who while working in East Africa noticed large tumors occurring in the jaws of children. Burkitt's lymphoma is much more common in Africa than the rest of the world. In Africa, where it is called endemic Burkitt's, it affects approximately 1 in 10,000 children and accounts for 50% of cancers seen in children in this part of the world. In the United States, Burkitt's lymphoma affects 1 in 400,000 children, accounting for approximately one third of all of the lymphomas seen in children. The lymphoma occurring in these cases is called sporadic Burkitt's lymphoma. When the pathologist examines these lymphomas under the microscope, instead of seeing the normal lymph node follicles or nodules, small, noncleaved lymphocytes are seen. In fact, another term used for these lymphomas is **small noncleaved cell lymphoma**. In Burkitt's-like lymphoma, larger cells are also seen. A characteristic finding under the microscope is the "starry sky" appearance that is a reflection of how rapidly the lymphoma cells are growing. The larger cells are macrophages that remove debris from the lymphoma cells that are dying.

Small noncleaved cell lymphoma

an aggressive, rapidly growing lymphoma.

The cause of these lymphomas, like all others, remains unknown, but the Epstein-Barr virus is involved. They occur more frequently in people with depressed immune systems, especially those infected with the HIV, the cause of AIDS. These associations suggest some role for an abnormality of the immune system in allowing these lymphomas to develop. An abnormality is also seen at the genetic level involving the lymphocytes of most patients with these lymphomas. A protein called c-Myc is produced in too great of a quantity and occurs because the gene that controls the production of this protein gets moved to a different chromosome where its production is continuously turned on. Too much of the protein drives the abnormal cell growth.

The most common way for Burkitt's lymphoma to present in African children is with swelling on one side of the jaw. It is usually a very rapidly growing tumor and can affect the upper or lower jaw or even both at the same time. Involvement of lymph nodes or bone marrow is uncommon. Involvement of the nervous system occurs more commonly than in the non-African type.

In both the sporadic Burkitt's and Burkitt's-like lymphomas, swelling of the jaw is uncommon. A mass in the abdomen occurs more frequently. Frequently, the bowel, pancreas, kidneys, and surrounding lymph nodes are involved. Involvement of the ovaries is common in females. Bone marrow involvement, which implies a poorer prognosis and also makes **central nervous system** involvement more likely, is unusual, occurring in 20% of patients. B symptoms do not occur frequently with this type of lymphoma. Another way for this type of lymphoma to present is with bone marrow and blood involvement, which is called **acute lymphoblastic leukemia**.

Central nervous system

the brain and spinal cord.

Acute lymphoblastic leukemia

a fast-growing type of leukemia.

40. What is lymphoblastic lymphoma?

Lymphoblastic lymphoma, another of the high-grade lymphomas, is more frequent in children than adults and accounts for one third of all lymphomas occurring in children but less than 5% of adult lymphomas. Most of these lymphomas (80%) are T-cell lymphomas, whereas the remainder are B-cell lymphomas. The pathologist is able to distinguish this type of lymphoma with a microscope. The lymphocytes appear very immature and can be stained for a particular enzyme, terminal deoxynucleotidyl transferase (EDT), which is not commonly seen with other types of lymphoma.

Lymphoblastic lymphoma occurs mostly in males and, when seen in adults, usually occurs between the ages of 20 to 30. It presents most frequently with a mass in the anterior mediastinum, the space in between the front of the lungs. Often, lymph nodes also occur in the neck or armpits. If the chest mass grows very quickly, it can cause pressure on the **trachea** (windpipe) or blood vessels. When this occurs, patients may complain of chest pain, shortness of breath, a choking sensation, headaches, or problems with vision. If a rapidly growing lymphoma causes these symptoms, treatment needs to begin immediately.

41. What lymphomas affect the skin?

Many lymphomas can affect the skin. If the skin is the only site affected, it is a primary cutaneous lymphoma. Secondary cutaneous lymphoma implies spread from other sites, such as lymph nodes. Although most lymphomas have the potential to involve skin, this is uncommon, and lymphoma involving the skin is usually primary. Most skin lymphomas are composed of T cells, but B-cell lymphomas also occur.

The skin can be affected in a number of ways, such as a small area of redness or skin thickening in one place such as on the forehead or scalp, or many small affected areas may occur in one region, eventually merging into one larger area. Often these areas are flat or only slightly raised off the surface, but sometimes actual nodules can appear. In some cases, the area can become very extensive. Patients often notice a skin abnormality that is changing and will see a dermatologist who may remove the lesion and send it to the laboratory for a pathologist's review. If a diagnosis of lymphoma is made, patients should be evaluated for any other evidence of lymphoma. Further tests may include a bone marrow examination and CT scans.

Mycosis fungoides, which is not uncommon, is a T-cell lymphoma that primarily affects the skin but occasionally can spread to the lymph nodes and bone marrow. It is more common in older individuals and causes a rash that can be very bothersome. Itchiness can be very severe. A number of treatment options are available, including **phototherapy**, chemotherapy skin treatments, and **interferon therapy** or **radiation therapy**. Newer medications, including bexarotene (Targretin) and denileukin diftitox (Ontak), are also effective.

Some lymphomas involving the skin are indolent and may not require any treatment; however, others are more aggressive, sometimes requiring an intravenous chemotherapy regimen such as cyclophosphamide, doxorubicin, vincristine, prednisone (often referred to by the acronym CHOP).

42. What are posttransplant lymphomas?

Posttransplant lymphoproliferative disorders frequently occur after a kidney, lung, or heart transplant but may occur after any type of organ transplant. They do occur after blood stem cell or marrow transplant, but this happens less frequently than after other types

Phototherapy
a type of therapy using UV light.

Interferon therapy
a type of immune therapy.

Radiation therapy
treatment using radiation.

Posttransplant lymphoproliferative disorders
a type of lymphoma that occurs after a transplant, usually because the immune system is depressed.

of transplant. Disorders appearing under the term posttransplant lymphoproliferative disorder can range from an abnormal growth of lymphocytes that is benign, resulting in lymph node enlargement that can be at one site or many sites throughout the body, to a very rapidly growing lymphoma that may involve the transplanted organ in addition to other parts of the body. Sometimes the lymphoma does not affect the lymph nodes in such cases.

Most of these lymphomas are associated with the Epstein-Barr virus, which can stimulate B lymphocytes to grow. It appears that people who have received a transplant and need to be kept on medication that suppresses the immune system so that the transplanted organ isn't rejected are particularly sensitive to Epstein-Barr virus infection. If Epstein-Barr virus infection occurs for the first time or if the virus is reactivated within the body in someone who was previously infected, a risk of developing the lymphoma exists (most of the adult population has been infected with Epstein-Barr virus, which often does not cause illness but stays dormant in the body). Fortunately, this only rarely occurs. It is estimated that 1% of kidney transplant recipients develop this type of lymphoma. The incidence is a little higher in heart and lung transplant recipients, possibly up to 6%. In bone marrow transplantation, the risk of posttransplant lymphoproliferative disorder increases if T cells are removed from the bone marrow graft. T cells are sometimes removed to try to prevent the complication of **graft versus host disease** (GVHD; see Question 88).

Graft versus host disease

an illness caused by the donor's immune system recognizing and attacking tissues and organs of the marrow recipient.

Treatment of this type of lymphoma is quite different than other lymphomas. The first step is to reduce the dose of the immune-suppressing anti-rejection drugs whenever possible. This is easier to do in patients with kidney transplants and also bone marrow transplants but is impossible in cases of a vital organ transplant such as the heart or lung. Patients may respond simply to withdrawal of these anti-rejection drugs. If further treatment is needed, chemotherapy may be used, and monoclonal antibodies such as Rituximab have also been shown to be useful. Clinical trials in bone marrow transplant recipients where T cells collected from the original bone marrow donor or even from normal individuals were administered to patients at risk of developing lymphoma have shown effectiveness in preventing posttransplant lymphoproliferative disorder. These treatments are also useful for the treatment of patients after they have developed posttransplant lymphoproliferative disorder.

HODGKIN'S LYMPHOMA

43. What are the different types of Hodgkin's disease?

Four main subtypes of Hodgkin's disease exist, and the pathologist distinguishes their appearance under a microscope. In Hodgkin's disease, unlike the non-Hodgkin's lymphomas, the malignant or cancerous cell may actually be difficult to find, as very few may be present and are greatly outnumbered by normal cells. The normal cells seen are those usually found in conditions of infection or inflammation. The number and types of the normal cells and the amount of scar tissue present in the lymph node will determine what type of Hodgkin's disease is present.

Nodular sclerosing Hodgkin's disease is the most common type, accounting for 75% of cases. It occurs

Nodular sclerosing Hodgkin's disease

the most common type of Hodgkin's disease.

more commonly in females and frequently involves the mediastinal lymph nodes, which are between the lungs. Commonly, neck lymph nodes will also be enlarged. When the biopsy specimen is examined under the microscope, thick bands of scar tissue (**fibrosis**) are seen surrounding the lymphocytes and inflammatory cells. Most patients have stage II disease at diagnosis, meaning at least two lymph node areas are involved on the same side of the diaphragm.

Fibrosis

the replacement of normal tissue with scar tissue.

Mixed cellularity Hodgkin's disease is another subtype. It is more common in men, can be quite aggressive at the time that it is diagnosed, and is frequently associated with bone marrow involvement; B symptoms are not uncommon.

Lymphocyte predominant Hodgkin's disease is also more common in men than women. This type of lymphoma may have the **CD20** protein on its surface. As a result, monoclonal antibodies such as Rituximab may have a role in treatment under some circumstances. The use of these monoclonal antibodies to treat Hodgkin's disease is currently experimental. This type of lymphoma can behave in an indolent fashion, similar to the indolent non-Hodgkin's lymphomas.

CD20

a protein on the surface of B lymphocytes and most B cell lymphomas.

The final and least common subtype is lymphocyte-depleted Hodgkin's disease, which generally behaves as a more aggressive type of lymphoma.

44. Can Hodgkin's disease turn into non-Hodgkin's lymphoma?

Some overlap exists between Hodgkin's disease and non-Hodgkin's lymphoma.

Some overlap exists between Hodgkin's disease and non-Hodgkin's lymphoma. The lymphocyte-predominant subtype has many similarities to indolent non-

Hodgkin's lymphoma, and features of both diseases may be present in the same patient. Occasionally, both Hodgkin's and non-Hodgkin's disease occur in the same patient at the same time. More commonly, however, a patient who had Hodgkin's disease at a younger age may subsequently develop non-Hodgkin's lymphoma. This second cancer may occur even 10 to 20 years after Hodgkin's disease was cured. Fortunately, this occurrence is quite rare.

Types of Lymphoma

PART FOUR

Staging and Treatment of Lymphoma

What happens after I'm told that I have lymphoma?

Should I get a second opinion?

More . . .

45. What happens after I'm told that I have lymphoma?

Hearing that you have lymphoma, as with any form of serious illness or cancer, can be a frightening and overwhelming experience. For most people, it is the first serious illness that they have faced, and many different emotions may arise. Patients often experience the various stages that are commonly associated with the grieving process, namely denial, anger, bargaining, depression, and finally acceptance. The duration and intensity of the different stages vary among individuals.

The surgeon who performed the biopsy is the first person to receive the results, which will be discussed with you at your first follow-up visit; however, many surgeons will not feel comfortable addressing the multitude of questions that are foremost in your mind. An appointment will be arranged with a lymphoma specialist, who can provide you with some answers. Whenever possible, this appointment should take place sooner rather than later to help minimize your anxiety.

A lymphoma specialist is a physician who is trained in hematology or oncology—and frequently both of these specialties. A hematologist has received specialty training in the management of blood disorders, including cancers related to the blood and lymphatic systems, such as lymphoma, leukemia, and multiple myeloma. An oncologist is a specialist that is trained in the management of all cancers in general. Most hematology and oncology training programs in the United States are combined, and as a result, most lymphoma patients receive treatment from a physician trained in both of these specialties. In communities with a university teaching hospital, there are often groups of physicians who specialize in mainly lymphoma or mainly leukemia.

As noted, the first step in coming to terms with the diagnosis is arming yourself with information and deciding on a plan of management. Therefore, hopefully your appointment with the lymphoma specialist can be expedited. For the first appointment, it is a good idea to bring your spouse, a close relative, or a friend to provide much needed emotional support, to remember to ask helpful questions, and to help in remembering the details. You may also find it helpful to tape record the meeting, as a lot information can be discussed at that first appointment. Before your appointment, your primary care doctor or surgeon will generally send or fax your medical records, including the biopsy results, to the lymphoma specialist's office. This allows your lymphoma doctor to review your information before the meeting. The benefit is that more time from the appointment can be dedicated to discussion about the nature of lymphoma, what other tests are needed, and how best to treat the disease. Your specialist will wish to review the symptoms that you have been experiencing and also obtain additional information about your past medical history. Because you have likely told the same story to a number of doctors and nurses previously, this can seem very repetitive; however, to ensure that nothing gets missed, this process is very important and is usually time well spent for both you and your new physician. This allows you and your doctor to get to know each other better.

At the initial visit, you may first meet with a nurse or medical assistant who will obtain some baseline infor-

The first step in coming to terms with the diagnosis is arming yourself with information and deciding on a plan of management.

Staging and Treatment of Lymphoma

mation. After filling out a form that provides details of your past medical and surgical history, family history, medications, and any drug allergies, you then will meet with the lymphoma doctor, who will ask questions about your symptoms and how you are currently feeling. You will then change into a gown to be examined. Gynecologic and rectal examinations are usually not required. The most important parts of the examination are the lymph nodes, liver, and spleen, but a general examination is also important in evaluating any other areas that the lymphoma may be affecting and what these effects might be, and also to get a sense of your overall health. This information is vital for deciding on the appropriate treatment. You may or may not prefer having your friend or relative remain in the room during the appointment or examination.

After the examination, your doctor will discuss lymphoma in general and your lymphoma in particular. Other required tests, including blood tests, scans, and usually a bone marrow examination, will give a complete picture of the extent of the lymphoma. A full discussion of the stage of the lymphoma and a treatment plan may need to wait for the next visit after the tests are completed. At that time, enough information will be available to allow for a more detailed discussion of your particular lymphoma. If possible, it is better not to discuss too much information at that first visit, especially if you are hearing the diagnosis for the first time. At the time of the next visit, your thinking can be much clearer, and you'll be able to absorb a lot more information. Your doctor may also be able to provide you with some reading material relating to lymphoma.

46. Should I get a second opinion?

A second opinion is a good idea if there is any doubt regarding the correct diagnosis, if you have any concerns about the proposed treatment, or if you do not feel good about your first lymphoma doctor. If there is doubt regarding the diagnosis, you may request that another pathologist reviews the slides. In most cases, however, the diagnosis is not in doubt, and often more than one pathologist within the department has already examined the slides. It can be comforting, however, to receive confirmation of the diagnosis and treatment options from another lymphoma specialist. Sometimes seeking a second opinion may result in transferring your care to the new doctor, depending on your preference and the options that your insurance company will allow. In any event, your first lymphoma doctor should be comfortable in having you seek a second opinion if you wish. Usually their office will give you a copy of all relevant material, including clinic notes and reports from the lymph node and bone marrow biopsies and any radiology studies, such as CT scans. The doctor who provides the second opinion will require these reports and will probably also need to have the actual biopsy slides and x-rays evaluated at the hospital to ensure that the advice given is based on accurate information.

It is important to recognize that there are many acceptable options and often more than one correct option for dealing with a diagnosis of lymphoma. You may, therefore, receive different recommendations from different physicians, with none of them being wrong. Some patients may then seek a third opinion, getting yet another set of recommendations. If you feel

It can be comforting, however, to receive confirmation of the diagnosis and treatment options from another lymphoma specialist.

comfortable with your first physician, second opinions may really be unnecessary and may lead to delays in proceeding with treatment as you attempt to sort all of the different options.

47. Apart from the biopsy, what other information is needed?

As mentioned previously, after the first time you see your lymphoma specialist, additional tests will need to be performed. These tests are needed to determine the answers to several questions: First, what is the stage of your lymphoma? This relates to which body parts are affected. CT scans to examine the lymph nodes in the chest, abdomen, and pelvis are often needed. A chest x-ray can be just as useful as a chest CT scan for the purpose of establishing the stage. A CT scan of the neck may also be obtained. A bone marrow biopsy is performed to evaluate the lymphoma at that site. Sometimes a bone marrow biopsy will be performed on both hips if the information makes a difference for treatment. Other tests performed less frequently include an MRI, a PET scan, or a gallium scan. These tests are discussed in Question 20 but can give you important information in some cases. Second, other tests can provide information on how your particular lymphoma is likely to progress—in other words, to determine the likely prognosis. Question 24 described how, in general, indolent lymphomas can be quite slow growing and can be managed with intermittent treatment over fairly long periods of time; however, this is true on average, and there may be certain features specific to your lymphoma that give a better idea of whether your lymphoma will be more or less aggressive. The features that are useful for determining the prognosis have been pooled together into a formula called the **International Prognostic Index** (IPI) (Question 48). All of this information will be available after the scans, blood tests, and bone marrow examination have been completed.

Other information needed will depend on your general health apart from the lymphoma. This information is important in determining your ability to tolerate the various treatment options. For example, your doctor may need to evaluate how well your heart is functioning, as some chemotherapy drugs used to treat lymphoma can affect heart function. If there is any concern about the ability of your heart to tolerate that treatment, an alternative chemotherapy drug may be chosen. Similarly, special breathing tests, called **pulmonary function tests**, may be required, as some drugs can cause lung damage. This damage may be worsened if your lung function is not optimal before beginning chemotherapy.

All of this information is generally obtained before starting treatment for the lymphoma. After the test results are available, your doctor will schedule another appointment to discuss the results and treatment plan with you.

48. What is the IPI?

The IPI is a method that is used to estimate a statistical chance of how well you will do with treatment. It was first introduced for intermediate-grade lymphoma but appears to be useful for most other types of non-Hodgkin's lymphomas. First introduced in 1993, it has gained wide acceptance as a very useful tool for planning treatment of lymphoma. In large studies from the

International Prognostic Index

a system to determine the prognosis of patients with lymphoma.

Pulmonary function tests

a set of tests performed to evaluate the ability of the lungs to function properly.

United States, Canada, and Europe, a number of features of the patients' lymphoma were documented and then correlated with the results of treatment. Certain of these features, when combined, allowed separation of patients into better and poorer prognosis groups. Another group with an intermediate prognosis was also identified.

Features helpful for determining prognosis were combined into this IPI: (1) age, (2) stage, (3) serum **lactate dehydrogenase**, (4) **performance status**, and (5) extranodal involvement. These features require further explanation. Older patients in general fare worse than younger ones; therefore, an age of older than 60 receives one point in the index. Second, patients with stage I or stage II disease generally do better than patients with stage III or stage IV disease; therefore, stage III or stage IV disease receives another point. The third feature is the level of a blood test, lactate dehydrogenase, which is present in red blood cells, liver, bone, and many other tissues. It is frequently increased in lymphoma patients and reflects the size of lymphoma and the rate at which it is growing. A level above normal is an additional risk factor and receives another point. Another point is given if the lymphoma involves sites other than the lymph nodes, including the bone marrow, the gut, liver, lung, and central nervous system (including the brain and spinal cord). The final feature in the IPI is the performance status, which is a measure of how well you are able to carry out your everyday activities. The Eastern Cooperative Oncology Group scale is shown in Table 6.

Other scoring systems, such as the **Karnofsky Performance Status scale**, are also used that evaluate the

Lactate dehydrogenase

an enzyme measured using a simple blood test.

Performance status

the level of ability with which patients can perform their routine daily activities.

Karnofsky Performance Status scale

a system to evaluate how patients do when performing the normal daily activities.

Table 6   Eastern Cooperative Oncology Group Performance Status Scale

0	No symptoms; fully active; able to carry out all normal activities.
1	Symptoms present but able to carry out normal activities; some difficulty with more strenuous activities.
2	Able to carry out normal self-care activities but limited in ability to work; up and about more than 50% of the time.
3	Capable of only limited self-care; confined to bed or chair more than 50% of waking hours.
4	Completely disabled; needing full-time assistance with normal self-care activities.

level of functioning. Another point is given for patients with a score of 2 to 4.

Thus, because there are five features in the IPI, any patient can have a score of 0 to 5, but most patients have a score of between 0 and 3. The score allows your doctor to estimate your likely response to treatment. The likelihood of success of the therapy is greatest with a lower score. Patients with higher scores may also do very well, as these likelihoods are statistical and may not apply to individual patients. If you are younger than age 60, the presence of lymphoma in sites other than the lymph nodes does not result in a worse prognosis. As a result, a modification to the IPI was made, resulting in the age-adjusted IPI. This relies on only three factors to determine the prognosis: stage, lactate dehydrogenase, and the performance status.

An example of how this information is important relates to decisions regarding treatment. If you have a higher score on the IPI, you may wish to consider other

treatments that may be available only through participation in a clinical trial. The IPI is also useful to ensure
that patients being treated in a clinical trial where two
treatments are being compared have similar characteristics. This ensures that any difference found between
the two treatments is related to the treatment and not
to differences in the patients that were treated in each
group. It is important to realize that the IPI was developed for the intermediate-grade lymphomas. It is often
applied to the indolent lymphomas but may not be as
useful in this setting. Also, the IPI attempts to predict
how patients with certain features receiving a CHOP-
like regimen will do. With improvements in
chemotherapy regimens, differences between patients
may not be so great, and, therefore, the IPI may be less
useful. One final note about these scores and prognostic indicators: You must always remember that they are
an estimate of how you might respond given your circumstances, and they are done for the sole purpose of
determining what sort of treatment could work best.
They do not in any way predict the future, nor are they
a statistic that dooms you to certain death or certain
recovery. Patients with a poor prognosis according to
these indicators often do survive lymphoma. It is
important that you do not "give up" simply because
you're facing a more daunting life-threatening challenge. Some of the more aggressive lymphomas are also
some of the most curable types of cancer. Survival
depends a great deal on determination to take your
treatment seriously and to work hard to maintain and
improve your health status. On the other hand, patients
with a good prognosis could misinterpret this estimate
as a guarantee of survival; if they do not pay close attention to their treatment regimen and overall health, they
could find themselves facing mortal illness. Thus, it is

*It is important
that you do
not "give up"
simply because
you're facing a
more daunting
life-threaten-
ing challenge.*

important to understand that these indicators are a guideline for treatment, not a crystal ball, and that you should not allow them to alter your determination to beat your lymphoma (Tables 7 and 8).

49. If I have Hodgkin's disease, does the IPI apply to me?

The IPI is not used for Hodgkin's disease. Instead, a number of other features relating to this type of lymphoma are useful for giving an indication of prognosis. This prognostic model was published in the *New England Journal of Medicine* in 1998, and factors shown to be important were being male, having stage IV disease, having a low level of **albumin** (a protein that a simple blood test measures), having anemia with a hemoglobin level of less than 10.5, having a white count above

Albumin

a special type of protein found in the bloodstream.

Table 7   IPI prognostic factors

- Age older than 60 years
- Eastern Cooperative Oncology Group performance score of 2 or more
- Elevated lactate dehydrogenase
- More than one site of extranodal involvement
- Stage III or stage IV lymphoma

Table 8   IPI risk categories

Risk Category	IPI Risk Factors
Low	0 or 1
Low–intermediate	2
High–intermediate	3
High	4 or 5

15,000, and, finally, having a low level of lymphocytes in the blood. As noted in the previous question, having a higher number of features does not necessarily signify a worse outcome. Treatment may be tailored differently to take into account a higher risk of relapse, and, again, patients with higher scores may benefit from seeking treatment in a clinical trial. Currently, trials are evaluating the use of stem cell transplantation as part of the initial treatment for patients with higher scores in both non-Hodgkin's lymphoma as well as Hodgkin's disease.

50. Are all types of lymphoma treated the same way?

No. Because there are many different types of lymphoma, the approach to treatment depends on whether the goal is cure or disease control. Even if the lymphoma is considered incurable, many different treatments are available that can control the lymphoma, often for very long periods of time. These treatments, given intermittently, can be very effective for disease control, keeping lymphoma patients feeling well often for many years. Especially in recent years, a large number of newer treatments have become available for lymphoma patients, and the outlook continues to improve at a rapid rate.

The approach to treatment depends on whether the goal is cure or disease control.

Newer techniques are becoming available to better distinguish between types of lymphoma that appear to be similar. Two patients may have a lymphoma that appears to be similar, yet with the same treatment they may respond quite differently. At least some of the explanation for this lies in differences in which proteins are being produced by the lymphoma cells. Certain proteins may cause a lymphoma to grow more rapidly or be resistant to a particular treatment. These proteins are determined by genes that can be turned on or off in lymphoma cells. Analyzing these genes can help to better determine the features of the lymphoma and, hopefully, to choose better treatments on the basis of this information. Gene Chip technology is the method used to evaluate which genes, and therefore which proteins, are turned on in lymphoma cells. It is currently a research technique, but many studies are clearly demonstrating its importance in the management of lymphoma. It will be very important in the near future for helping to choose the correct treatment for different patients who appear to have the same type of lymphoma.

51. What treatments are available for lymphoma?

Treatments used for lymphoma include chemotherapy, radiation therapy, and more recently, **biologic therapy**. Chemotherapy refers to the use of drugs, usually given by mouth or in a vein (intravenously). After administration, the chemotherapy enters the bloodstream and travels to every part of the body. It can be given either as one drug alone (single-agent chemotherapy) or combined with other chemotherapy drugs (combination chemotherapy). A perfect chemotherapy drug would damage only cancer cells, but most of these drugs in use today can also damage normal cells. Chemotherapy can be given in very high doses, but the side effect of this is often destruction of the bone marrow. Giving high-dose chemotherapy along with the infusion of bone marrow stem cells is the basis for bone marrow or **stem cell transplantation** (discussed

Biologic therapy
treatment that uses the body's immune responses to attack diseased cells.

Stem cell transplantation
the procedure of replacing bone marrow stem cells to allow recovery of blood cells after high-dose chemotherapy.

in Questions 81 and 82). Radiation, another type of treatment, is usually given to specific areas of the body in which the lymphoma is involved to control disease at that location. It treats the lymphoma that is only in the area that gets treated. Sometimes it is used in an attempt to prevent the lymphoma from coming back at a particular site after treatment with chemotherapy.

Biologic therapy is actually a vague term that implies the use of many different types of treatments. In common, they are all specifically designed to take advantage of new knowledge of the biology of lymphoma and the immune system. Such biologic therapy can include **antibody therapy** and vaccine therapy.

Antibody therapy
the use of antibodies
to treat cancer.

52. How is indolent lymphoma treated?

After diagnosis and staging, the next very important step is to make decisions about treatment. As strange as it may seem, one of the options is something called "watch and wait." Other options include low doses of chemotherapy pills, more intensive intravenous chemotherapy, antibody therapy, and transplant options. All of these options are acceptable depending on the specific features of an individual patient's lymphoma and also on the patient's personal preferences. You can discuss with your lymphoma doctor the merits of each of these approaches.

The "watch-and-wait" concept has been around for many years and arose from observations that the indolent lymphomas often are slow growing, that frequently they are not associated with any symptoms, and that they can generally be controlled with therapy when necessary. Earlier treatment has not been shown to prolong survival. Furthermore, as some treatments can have long-term harmful effects, saving their use for later when they may be needed more urgently helps to minimize this. Also, accepting watch and wait carries with it the understanding that the indolent lymphomas are not curable. Additional reasons to consider the watch-and-wait approach are possible side effects from chemotherapy and also that the chemotherapy drugs work best the first time that they are used. Therefore, keeping the drugs in reserve until symptoms or problems occur or seem likely to occur may be a valid strategy. Not every patient is comfortable with this approach, and indeed, some physicians feel that this is a "defeatist" attitude. Certainly, if you feel uncomfortable with this approach, you should discuss your feelings with your physician or obtain a second opinion. If symptoms are present or if the lymph node enlargement is causing problems, treatment will be recommended.

When watch and wait is acceptable, the lymphoma specialist should regularly see his or her patients. You should be alert for any symptoms that could indicate progression of lymphoma. Blood counts should be checked regularly, because any fall in the blood counts could signal disease progression. Occasionally, patients may go for many years without requiring treatment. Most patients, however, need some form of treatment after a few months to 2 years. For many patients and also some doctors, the idea of watch and wait is objectionable. Patients often prefer to be proactive and to feel in control as much as possible. These are valid reasons to choose treatment over watch and wait. Some of the arguments used to support watch and wait may not apply to the newer treatment options that have become available over the past few years. Whether earlier treatment with such agents can improve survival remains to be demonstrated in clinical trials.

Table 9   Options available for the treatment of indolent lymphoma

Watch and wait

Chemotherapy pills

Intravenous chemotherapy in combination

Localized radiation (rarely)

Monoclonal antibody therapy (e.g., rituximab [Rituxan™])

Radioimmunotherapy (e.g., ibritumomab tiuxetan [Zevalin™])

Autologous stem cell transplant

Allogeneic stem cell transplant

If the decision is made to proceed with treatment, many options are available (shown in Table 9).

Traditionally, chemotherapy is the first treatment that most patients with indolent lymphoma receive. The challenge is to select the right agent or combination of agents best suited to the patient's circumstances (specific chemotherapy drugs are discussed in Question 59). The approach to treating indolent lymphoma differs among physicians. Often there is no one right way to treat an individual patient, and a staged approach is taken. With this strategy, the mildest chemotherapy that is likely to produce a response is the first chemotherapy chosen. This may take the form of pills, as in chlorambucil (leukeran) given with or without the steroid prednisone. If the lymphoma responds but requires further treatment at a later time, a combination regimen, such as cyclophosphamide, vincristine, and prednisone (CVP), may be given. The next time that treatment is required, the CHOP regimen is given. The rationale for this staged approach is to use less chemotherapy early, when the lymphoma is the most responsive to chemotherapy. Over time, the lymphoma is likely to be more resistant to chemotherapy, and stronger regimens will be needed. Giving stronger chemotherapy earlier has not been shown to prolong survival over milder chemotherapy and may add additional side effects that may cause more serious problems in later years or may interfere with quality of life.

On the other hand, many physicians feel that a more intensive treatment, although more likely to cause side effects, will produce a longer remission. This may allow patients to go longer before needing another type of treatment. One downside of this is that it is unlikely that after receiving the more intensive treatments the patients will subsequently respond to less intensive treatments. Certain patients will benefit from the less intensive treatments, often for many years, and the IPI may allow such patients to be identified, thereby sparing them overly aggressive treatments. The CHOP-like regimens should generally be reserved for patients with indolent lymphoma with a more aggressive presentation or for patients who progress after treatment with less intensive treatments.

Fludarabine is another useful drug if you have indolent lymphoma. It is often used for the progression of the lymphoma occurring after treatment with CHOP. The CHOP regimen may not be recommended for some patients because of its effect on heart function; fludarabine may thus be a good choice for these patients. Because fludarabine depresses the immune system, you need to be especially watchful for any signs of infection.

The newest treatments for indolent lymphoma are the monoclonal antibody rituximab (Rituxan™) and its relative, ibritumomab tiuxetan (Zevalin™), which carries a radioactive molecule to the lymphoma. The availability of these antibody treatments is dramatically changing the way that many types of lymphoma are treated. The Food and Drug Administration currently approved rituximab for treatment of patients who progress after receiving chemotherapy, but newer clinical trials are demonstrating that it is an effective drug when used even as the first treatment for indolent lymphoma. Rituximab can also safely be combined with many chemotherapy regimens to improve the results over the use of chemotherapy alone. Very intensive chemotherapy with or without radiation is also an option for some patients. Because these high doses can destroy the patient's own bone marrow, they are given in conjunction with an **autologous stem cell transplant** (discussed in Questions 81 and 82). The higher treatment doses may result in a longer remission in certain patients, but, unfortunately, this strategy does not offer a cure.

Autologous stem cell transplant

a transplant where you are your own bone marrow stem cells donor.

A different type of transplant, and the only treatment option that can potentially cure indolent lymphoma, is an allogeneic transplant, which uses bone marrow stem cells from a brother or sister or sometimes from an unrelated individual. Because there are significant risks associated with an allogeneic transplant, it is not a suitable treatment option for many patients with indolent lymphoma.

Radiation therapy may be another useful option for the treatment of indolent lymphoma. Occasionally, patients may have stage I or II disease with one or two lymph nodes areas involved. In such cases, especially in the rare situation of stage I indolent lymphoma, radiation may actually be a cure. If not a cure, it may actually delay the lymphoma from returning for many years.

53. How does my doctor know what treatment to recommend for my low-grade lymphoma?

Your lymphoma specialist will make a recommendation for treatment after reviewing all aspects of your particular lymphoma and your general state of health. This is important in determining your ability to tolerate the different chemotherapy drugs or combination regimens. Your doctor's experience in treating other patients with similar types of lymphoma, knowledge gained from reading the medical literature, continuing medical education (attending lectures or conferences), and discussions with colleagues all provide the background for making treatment recommendations. Many centers, especially the larger cancer centers, have a number of lymphoma specialists who discuss all of the new cases of lymphoma at a weekly conference. Discussions from these meetings can be very helpful when deciding on a treatment plan. Pathologists and radiologists will often also be at this meeting; thus, all aspects of the case can be considered together. The discussion can also serve to provide you with a number of second opinions.

It can be quite frustrating when your physician presents a number of different treatment options and asks you to decide which treatment to receive. Given that many options may be "right," you may need assistance in this decision; thus, you should ask your doctor for further guidance in making the best decision.

54. How is intermediate-grade lymphoma treated?

Because intermediate-grade lymphoma is an aggressive type of lymphoma that can be cured in many cases, the approach to treatment is therefore very different than with the indolent lymphomas, because treatment can often be delayed until the time of progression; however, intermediate-grade lymphomas are frequently fast growing, requiring treatment soon after diagnosis. Because many patients can be cured, the approach involves giving the treatment that is the most likely to result in a cure as the initial therapy. For many years, CHOP has been the best treatment for intermediate-grade lymphoma and continues to be the most commonly used chemotherapy regimen for the aggressive lymphomas. Many similar chemotherapy regimens have been compared with CHOP, but none have proven to be better. Overall, approximately 40 to 50% of patients will be cured with CHOP. The IPI is helpful in determining this, but you should remember that many patients with higher IPI scores can still do well, especially with some of the newer treatments now available. After the diagnosis and staging have been completed, most patients receive six to eight cycles of chemotherapy. CHOP is given every 3 weeks, indicating that one cycle lasts 3 weeks. Six cycles of chemotherapy, when given on time every 3 weeks, take 18 weeks to complete.

Fewer cycles of CHOP can safely be given if the lymphoma is stage I or stage II. Essentially, only three cycles of CHOP need be given instead of six to eight cycles, but only if radiation therapy is given to the one or two areas involved by the lymphoma. Studies have demonstrated that three cycles of chemotherapy followed by radiation are equivalent to six to eight cycles of chemotherapy in stage I or stage II intermediate-grade lymphoma. Patients are therefore exposed to less chemotherapy, and the entire treatment course is shorter, resulting in fewer complications from the treatment. Whether you can receive radiation and therefore be spared the extra cycles of chemotherapy depends on where the lymphoma is in your body. In some cases, it may be too risky to radiate particular areas of the body, and your doctor may prefer to administer six cycles of chemotherapy.

Some patients, even though they receive six to eight cycles of chemotherapy, may still need radiation, especially if the site of lymphoma is bulky. Radiation to bulky sites that were present before chemotherapy, even if they have disappeared with treatment, may help prevent the lymphoma from returning. Recently, studies have shown that the cure rate may be better if the monoclonal antibody Rituximab (Rituxan) is given along with CHOP. Significantly better outcomes have been reported for patients who are older than 60 years who received CHOP plus Rituximab. Studies are currently under way to determine whether this is also true in patients who are less than 60 years old.

55. Is intermediate-grade lymphoma curable if it returns after therapy?

If your lymphoma returns after chemotherapy, a realistic chance of cure is still possible. High-dose chemotherapy with an autologous stem cell transplant is the most accepted treatment for people in otherwise

If your lymphoma returns after chemotherapy, a realistic chance of cure is still possible.

good general health. In order to determine whether patients are likely to respond to the high-dose chemotherapy and transplant, another chemotherapy regimen is first given to shrink the lymphoma. If the lymphoma responds to this treatment, it is likely that a transplant is indicated. If your doctor is considering a transplant at this time, it is a good idea for you to be referred to a transplant center, where a transplant physician can determine whether you are likely to derive benefit from the transplant; if so, a number of tests to evaluate your heart, kidney, and lung functions and your general ability to withstand the transplant will be required. These tests should be performed as you are receiving your chemotherapy so that there is no delay between the chemotherapy and proceeding to the transplant. Of all patients who respond to the salvage chemotherapy and go on to receive an autologous transplant, approximately 35 to 40% will be cured. Many others may receive a benefit in terms of a longer period before the lymphoma returns. The chances of cure without a transplant in this setting are much smaller. The most common salvage chemotherapy regimens contain a chemotherapy drug called platinum. They include the ESHAP, ICE, and DHAP regimens, which are usually given two or three times at 3- to 4-week intervals for ESHAP and DHAP and every 2 weeks for ICE. If you are responding, a transplant may be proposed. ESHAP and DHAP cycles are given 3 to 4 weeks apart, whereas ICE is given every 2 weeks. Clinical trials are evaluating whether adding the monoclonal antibody Rituximab to the chemotherapy can produce better results than chemotherapy alone.

56. How is high-grade lymphoma treated?

The high-grade lymphomas can also be cured, in many cases, with chemotherapy. These are generally more rapidly growing than the other types of lymphoma, and, as a result, treatment is more urgent. The treatment regimens used for these lymphomas consist of a large number of different chemotherapy drugs given at frequent intervals. Patients usually require hospitalization for the few days each month when the chemotherapy is administered. These regimens are similar to the treatments used for childhood leukemia. Because most of these lymphomas are very fast growing, they can also be very sensitive to the effects of chemotherapy; therefore, there is a very high rate of complete response. The lymph nodes can shrink very fast, often over a period of days. As the cancer cells die, they release a lot of different toxic substances into the bloodstream. The kidneys need to remove these toxins from the body or serious problems can arise, including kidney failure. Intravenous fluids are given in large quantities, and the medication allopurinol is given to help the kidneys cope. Sodium bicarbonate is often also given, as the kidneys do a better job at a higher pH.

Once a remission is achieved, further therapy is given to prevent the lymphoma from returning. More cycles of the same or similar chemotherapy may be given. The number of cycles varies, as there are a number of different regimens available. Some clinical trials are evaluating the addition of monoclonal antibodies to the chemotherapy.

An important aspect to treating this type of lymphoma is the central nervous system. This type of lymphoma has a higher possibility of central nervous system involvement. In order to evaluate the central nervous system, a **spinal tap** (lumbar puncture) is performed. The **spinal fluid** is analyzed for any lymphoma cells, and often, at the same time, a small amount of chemotherapy is given through the spinal needle into the spinal fluid (**intrathecal**). The chemotherapy then circulates through the spinal fluid, including the fluid around the brain. Giving this dose of chemotherapy before knowing whether the lymphoma involves the central nervous system does no harm. If there is central nervous system lymphoma, more intrathecal chemotherapy and possibly radiation will be necessary. Even if there is no lymphoma present in the spinal fluid, many patients also need further intrathecal chemotherapy to prevent lymphoma from occurring at this site.

In some patients, especially if the lymphoma recurs after a complete treatment course, an autologous stem cell transplant may be required and can result in a cure.

57. How is Hodgkin's disease treated?

The chance of being cured from Hodgkin's disease is overall approximately 60 to 80%, making Hodgkin's disease the most curable of all of the lymphomas. In order to understand the treatment of Hodgkin's disease, it is important to realize that it tends to spread from one lymph node area to other lymph node areas close by as it progresses. The non-Hodgkin's lymphomas do not have this tendency; instead, they often skip areas. As a result, the stage of Hodgkin's disease is the most important factor in deciding on treatment. Previously, physicians used to go to great lengths to determine the stage. An operation called a "staging laparotomy" was per-

Spinal tap

the procedure for obtaining a sample of spinal fluid.

Spinal fluid

the fluid surrounding the brain and spinal fluid.

Intrathecal

an injection into the fluid surrounding the spinal cord or brain.

formed if the lymphoma appeared to involve only one or two areas. This operation involved making an incision in the abdomen, taking small pieces (biopsies) of the liver and any lymph nodes, and also removing the spleen. This operation was done to be absolutely certain that the lymphoma was in only one or two areas. If this was the case, radiation treatment alone could be given rather than chemotherapy, since it would then result in a high chance of cure and would avoid any chemotherapy-related complications. This operation is rarely needed today.

Currently, Hodgkin's disease that is stage I or stage II is generally treated with radiation therapy alone. In most cases, this is curative. Certain features, however, make it likely that you also will need chemotherapy given before the radiation. Question 48 discusses the features that are higher risk, as these often suggest the need for chemotherapy. Also, patients with B symptoms also need chemotherapy. In some cases, less chemotherapy can be used in patients who are receiving both chemotherapy and radiation than in patients receiving chemotherapy alone.

If the higher risk features are not present, radiation alone can be given. If the Hodgkin's lymphoma is stage III or stage IV, chemotherapy is usually the best option. Most patients with Hodgkin's disease receive the ABVD chemotherapy regimen, which has been used throughout the 1990s. Starting in the early 1960s, the MOPP chemotherapy regimen was found to be very useful. The ABVD chemotherapy regimen is perhaps slightly more effective than MOPP, but has fewer side effects. Whereas MOPP was associated with a high rate of infertility, fertility is maintained in most patients after ABVD. Also, after MOPP there is a higher rate of other cancers, including leukemia. This is not the case with ABVD.

The drugs in the ABVD regimen are given every 2 weeks, and one cycle lasts 1 month. Six to eight cycles are usually required.

A newer regimen termed Stanford V appears to be an effective treatment for many patients with Hodgkin's disease. It takes only 12 weeks to complete and is currently being compared to ABVD in clinical trials. Radiation therapy is a component of this treatment.

PART FIVE

Chemotherapy and Radiation Therapy

What is chemotherapy?

What chemotherapy drugs are used to treat lymphoma?

More . . .

58. What is chemotherapy?

Paul Erlich (1854–1915) introduced the concept of chemotherapy. His revolutionary idea was to use mice to test antibiotics for activity against infectious disease. Subsequently, mice with tumors were used to test the activity of other chemicals against cancer. Further advances in the development of chemotherapy were made during World War I. Mustard gas was being tested as a chemical weapon, and exposure to this agent led to shrinkage of lymph nodes and bone marrow. These observations led to the use of nitrogen mustard for the treatment of lymphoma in the early 1940s.

"Chemotherapy" actually means the treatment of disease with any drug. However, in common usage, it refers to the treatment of cancer using drugs. Chemotherapy drugs are the most widely used treatments used for lymphoma. Many different types of chemotherapy drugs are available, and new ones are continuously being developed. Many are derived from natural products found in the environment. The National Cancer Institute has a specific program in which scientists all over the world obtain samples from plants, trees, ocean-dwelling creatures, and so forth, and test them in the laboratory for any activity against cancer.

Chemotherapy drugs are given either orally or intravenously, or, less commonly, are injected directly into a muscle (**intramuscular**), under the skin (**subcutaneous**), or into the spinal fluid surrounding the brain and spinal cord (intrathecal). However the drugs are given, apart from intrathecal, the chemotherapy gets into the bloodstream and is distributed to all parts of the body. This type of treatment is referred to as **systemic treatment** and is different from **local treatment**,

Systemic treatment

a treatment such as chemotherapy that reaches all body parts through the bloodstream.

in which a specific site is targeted. Examples of local treatment include radiation and surgery. The benefit of chemotherapy over surgery or radiation is its ability to reach all parts of the lymphatic system. Depending on the specific type of lymphoma, even if lymph nodes in other areas are not enlarged, they may still be affected at the microscopic level and, therefore, benefit from chemotherapy. Surgery or radiation will not be helpful against these areas of microscopic involvement. Most chemotherapy drugs kill the more rapidly dividing cells. Lymphoma cells divide more rapidly than normal cells, especially the intermediate- and high-grade lymphomas. This explains their better response to chemotherapy than the indolent lymphomas. It also explains why chemotherapy affects the bone marrow, the lining of the gut, and eggs and sperm more than slower dividing cells.

Chemotherapy drugs are classified into groups based on their exact mechanism of action on cell machinery. Different groups of drugs act at different phases of the cell life cycle. Drugs acting on different mechanisms within cancer cells are often used together as "combination chemotherapy regimens," having a greater effect against the cancer than single drugs.

59. What chemotherapy drugs are used to treat lymphoma?

Many chemotherapy drugs are used to treat lymphoma. The number of available agents has increased, especially in the past few years. Newer drugs such as monoclonal antibodies have been made available recently and have the potential to increase the activity of chemotherapy drugs against lymphoma. Clinical studies continue to

Local treatment
treatment aimed at a particular area of the body. For example, radiation treatment is local whereas chemotherapy is systemic.

Chemotherapy and Radiation Therapy

demonstrate better ways to use and combine the chemotherapy drugs that have been available for many years. Chemotherapy drugs can be used either alone or in combination, and they are usually given orally as pills or intravenously. When given intravenously, they can be given as a **bolus** (a quick injection), a short infusion, or a continuous infusion (Table 10).

Chlorambucil and cyclophosphamide have been available for many years, both belonging to a class of chemotherapy drugs called **alkylating agents**, which were the first chemotherapy drugs demonstrated to have anticancer activity in humans. During World War I, sulfur mustard gas was used as a weapon and was noted to produce **aplasia,** or shrinkage of lymph tissue. Subsequently, the related nitrogen mustards, which lacked the gases' nasty effects on the lungs and the skin, were examined for activity against lymphoma. Nitrogen mustard was developed as a result of such studies. Subsequently, other less toxic but more effective alkylating agents have been introduced. Chlorambucil and cyclophosphamide are currently the most commonly used alkylating agents that are used to treat lymphoma. Alkylating agents cause cross-linking of DNA, adding an extra chemical group to the DNA strands. This prevents the cell from dividing, which is necessary for its normal growth. Without the ability to divide, the cell dies.

Chlorambucil (Leukeran) is taken orally and is usually given for 5 days every month or once every 2 weeks. It is generally well tolerated but can produce an upset stomach, which can be prevented with antinausea medication. It does not usually cause hair loss (**alopecia**). Its main side effect is to suppress the bone mar-

Bolus
a rapid administration of an intravenous injection.

Alkylating agents
a class of chemotherapy drugs.

Aplasia
a condition in which blood cells are not produced.

Alopecia
hair loss.

Table 10   Standard chemotherapy regimens for lymphoma

Chemotherapy Drugs and Combinations	How Given
Chlorambucil with or without prednisone	Orally or intravenously
Cyclophosphamide (C)	Orally
Vincristine (O or V)	Intravenously
Prednisone (P)	Orally
Fludarabine	Intravenously
Cyclophosphamide (C)	Intravenously
Doxorubicin (H)	Intravenously
Vincristine (O)	Intravenously
Prednisone (P)	Orally
Fludarabine (F)	Intravenously
Cyclophosphamide (C)	Intravenously
Fludarabine (F)	Intravenously
Mitoxantrone (N)	Intravenously
Dexamethasone (D)	Intravenously
Cyclophosphamide (C)	Intravenously
Mitoxantrone (N)	Intravenously
Vincristine (O)	Intravenously
Prednisone (P)	Orally
Ifosfamide (I)	Intravenously
Carboplatin (C)	Intravenously
Etoposide (E)	Intravenously
Etoposide (E)	Intravenously
Solumedrol (S)	Intravenously
Ara-C (HA)	Intravenously
Cisplatinum (P)	Intravenously
Rituximab (R)	Intravenously
Rituximab + CHOP	Intravenously
Rituximab + other chemotherapy	Intravenously

Chemotherapy and Radiation Therapy

row, which is seen as a drop in the white blood cell count and the platelet count. The maximal drop in the counts occurs at 3 to 4 weeks, and weekly blood counts are generally obtained to monitor the blood counts. Chlorambucil combined with prednisone may produce a slightly faster response than chlorambucil alone but does not have any other benefit.

Cyclophosphamide (Cytoxan) can be given intravenously or orally. For the treatment of indolent lymphoma, it is usually given orally as part of the CVP regimen. It is given for 5 days every 3 weeks. It may cause some nausea and vomiting, which can be controlled with antinausea medicine, and frequently causes hair loss. Over a prolonged period, it may cause bleeding from damage to the lining of the bladder. Cyclophosphamide also affects the blood counts. A drop in the white blood cell count is usually seen (greatest at 10 to 14 days).

Chlorambucil and CVP produce similar results. Responses may occur faster with CVP, but this is only an advantage if you have bothersome symptoms needing a more rapid response. Many patients prefer chlorambucil because it is taken by mouth and does not cause hair loss.

An important consideration when taking alkylating agents is the risk of second cancers. The risk for developing leukemia is estimated at approximately 6% and emphasizes the need to consider possible long-term complications of any treatment, especially for somebody without symptoms.

Another chemotherapy drug commonly used for the treatment of lymphoma is doxorubicin (Adriamycin), which belongs to a class of drugs called the antitumor antibiotics. They also cause cancer cells to die by interfering with the DNA. Mitoxantrone (Novantrone) is a similar drug. Doxorubicin is generally combined with cyclophosphamide, vincristine, and prednisone in the CHOP regimen. If mitoxantrone (Novantrone) is used instead of doxorubicin, it is called CNOP. CHOP is the most commonly used regimen for the intermediate-grade lymphomas, but is also frequently used as a treatment option for indolent lymphomas. It is administered every 3 weeks. Therefore, one cycle is 3 weeks in length, and six to eight cycles are usually given.

Side effects of doxorubicin also include bone marrow suppression. The lowest blood counts are at 10 to 14 days. Nausea and vomiting are usually preventable with premedication, and hair loss also occurs. Doxorubicin can also occasionally produce heart muscle damage and with prolonged treatment may even produce heart failure. Because of this small risk, a measurement of heart function is often obtained before starting the CHOP regimen. As initial therapy for indolent lymphoma, CHOP does not appear to be better than chlorambucil or CVP in terms of lengthening overall years of life, but it produces a more rapid response and maybe a higher chance of a complete response. In certain cases, it may offer significant advantages over other treatments.

Fludarabine (Fludara) is another important drug in the treatment of lymphoma. It belongs to a class of drugs called nucleoside analogues. Fludarabine is taken up into lymphocytes and blocks the activity of an enzyme important for lymphocyte growth. It is quite active against cells that divide only slowly, including the indolent lymphomas.

Fludarabine is given as an intravenous infusion over 30 minutes, generally for 5 days in a row every month (each cycle being 1 month) for a variable number of cycles, depending on how well the patient responds. Some nausea or vomiting may occur but is unusual. Bone marrow suppression occurs, resulting in the need to monitor blood counts regularly. Fludarabine is also quite effective at killing normal lymphocytes, and this can be a very long-lasting effect. As a result, patients are at higher risk of developing certain infections such as shingles or even *Pneumocystis carinii pneumoniae*, an infection more commonly seen in individuals with AIDS. The antibiotic septra (Bactrim) is very effective at preventing *Pneumocystis carinii pneumoniae* when given twice a week.

An oral form of fludarabine is available in some countries outside of the United States. It appears to be as effective as the intravenous form and hopefully will be available some time in the near future in this country.

Fludarabine has been administered in combination with other chemotherapy drugs such as cyclophosphamide and mitoxantrone. The combination may have advantages in certain individuals, but the incidence of side effects is greater.

Vincristine (Oncovin) and vinblastine (Velban) belong to a class of drugs called the vinca alkaloids. The vinca alkaloids inhibit cancer cells by binding to **microtubules**, which prevent the cell from dividing normally. Both drugs are given intravenously and usually are part of a combination chemotherapy regimen. Vincristine is the V in the CVP regimen and also the O in the CHOP regimen. Vinblastine is used more commonly in Hodgkin's disease.

Microtubules

structures present in individual cells that are important for allowing cells to divide.

Hair loss may occur with both drugs, although more commonly with vincristine. The main side effect of vincristine is mild nerve damage. This is quite common, and the frequency increases with ongoing treatment. Often the first thing noticed is tingling in the fingers and toes. It is important at clinic visits to tell your physician about these changes. Jaw pain may also occur because the drug affects nerves in that area. Constipation as a result of vincristine affecting the nerves of the gut is also common, and, if necessary, you should take a stool softener or a laxative to prevent this complication. The nerve damage that vincristine causes is generally reversible. Your doctor may reduce the dose or stop the drug completely depending on your symptoms, which generally improve after the drug is discontinued but may take many months to return to normal.

Etoposide (VePesid or VP-16) kills lymphoma cells by interacting with a protein that is important for stabilizing DNA.

Ifosfamide and carboplatin are active in lymphoma. These drugs are often used together with etoposide in the ICE regimen. Ifosfamide belongs to the same class as cyclophosphamide and has a similar side effect profile. Carboplatin is a similar drug to cisplatinum, but its main side effect is bone marrow suppression.

60. How is chemotherapy given?

Most patients with lymphoma receive chemotherapy intravenously. Other ways to administer the drugs include by mouth, under the skin, into the muscle, or into the CSF (intrathecal).

If a number of cycles of chemotherapy are to be given intravenously, one very useful item is an **indwelling**

Indwelling catheter

an intravenous catheter that can remain in place for longer periods than a few days.

Hickman catheter

an intravenous line that passes through the skin into a large vein near the heart. It provides a safer and easier way to administer chemotherapy and obtain blood samples.

Broviac catheter

a type of catheter that goes directly into a large vein to allow easier administration of medications and blood tests.

catheter. Having a catheter can simplify the process of receiving chemotherapy infusions or injections. Indwelling catheters are essentially hollow tubes, one end of which is placed into a vein close to the heart. The other end of the tube is conveniently located under the skin or actually comes out through the skin where it is available fifth connection to the chemotherapy bag. This prevents needing to find a vein and inserting a new intravenous needle each time that chemotherapy is given. It is also a safer way to administer chemotherapy. The catheters are also useful for taking blood samples. Blood transfusions, antibiotics, or intravenous fluids can also be given through the catheter.

Several different types of indwelling catheters exist and can remain in place for many months or even a year or more. Two main types of catheter exist and differ depending on whether it is entirely under the skin, as in the case of the "Portacath," or if a part of it comes out through the skin (Figure 3).

The first type of catheter is a **Hickman** or **Broviac** catheter. Part of it is external, with approximately 6 inches of tubing outside the skin. This catheter

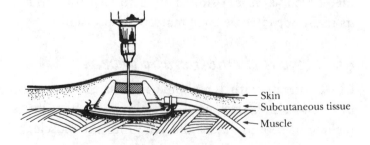

Skin
Subcutaneous tissue
Muscle

Figure 3   Schematic drawing of an implantable port. Reprinted from Yarbro CH, Frogge MH, Goodman M, Groenwald SL: *Cancer Nursing: Principles and Practice*, Fifth Ed. Copyright © 2000, Jones and Bartlett Publishers, Inc.

requires dressing changes, and the tubes need to be flushed daily with a medication to keep blood from clotting in it. The patient can be taught to do this at home. The second type of catheter is a port or Porta-cath, which remains entirely under the skin without any external component. It does not require any dressing and requires only monthly flushing. The flushing requires the services of a nurse, and each time the port is accessed, it requires that a needle be inserted through the skin. In the case of both catheters, the part that is accessed for chemotherapy is usually placed on the upper part of the chest, in the front. Smaller catheters may also be useful in some situations and may be placed in the arms instead of the chest wall, such as the percutaneous implantable central catheter or PICC (Figure 4).

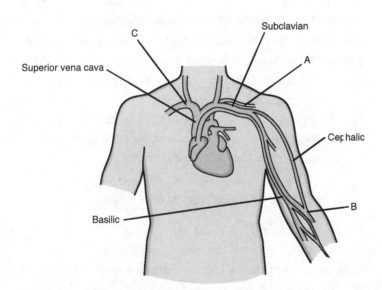

Figure 4   Sites of catheter placement: (A) percutaneous central venous catheters; (B) PICC lines; (C) Hickman-type catheters, Groshongs. The catheter placements indicated by (A) and (C) can be in the subclavian vein on either side; the access for the catheter is usually placed in the upper chest wall and tunnelled under the skin to the point of insertion into the vein.

61. What problems can result from having a catheter?

Side effects from catheters do occur, but in most patients the convenience and comfort of a catheter outweigh its risks. A surgeon or an **interventional radiologist** (a doctor who performs surgical procedures such as placing an intravenous catheter using x-ray equipment) places these catheters, usually using local anesthesia. Complications rarely occur at the time that a catheter is first placed but include bleeding that is usually easily controlled. More seriously, but quite rarely, a lung can be punctured. Symptoms of a punctured lung include shortness of breath, cough, and chest pain. If there is any doubt, your doctor will obtain a chest x-ray.

Interventional radiologist

a physician who is trained in using X-rays to aid in the performance of some types of surgical procedures, such as placing catheters.

Complications that may develop during the time a catheter is in place can include infection or a blood clot forming around the catheter. Thus, some doctors place patients on a low dose of coumadin, a blood thinner, in an attempt to prevent blood clots.

If you want an indwelling catheter and your healthcare team recommends this approach, you can discuss which catheter is the most appropriate.

62. What are the side effects of chemotherapy?

In this question, we discuss general side effects that may occur with most chemotherapy drugs. The extent of side effects varies depending on the specific drugs that you receive, how they are administered, and how your body reacts to them. Your doctor and nurse will explain the side effects that you are most likely to

The extent of side effects of chemotherapy varies.

experience. Most people associate nausea, vomiting, and hair loss with chemotherapy, but this is variable from person to person depending on the chemotherapy regimen. Today, good drugs are available to prevent nausea and vomiting. Thus, if you experience nausea or vomiting the first time that you receive chemotherapy, ask your physician whether any changes can be made for future treatments.

Most chemotherapy drugs kill some normal cells as well as lymphoma cells. Some of the side effects that you experience result from damage to these normal cells. The normal cells that are the most affected are those in areas where cells grow and divide most rapidly. These areas include hair follicles, bone marrow, the **gastrointestinal tract**, and the **reproductive system**. Thus, the most common side effects are hair loss, mouth sores, diarrhea, and problems related to infertility, although you should remember that having had chemotherapy does not necessarily mean that you are infertile. Because most chemotherapy drugs have severe effects on sperm and eggs, it is very important not to conceive while receiving chemotherapy. Appropriate contraception practices should be used if there is any potential for pregnancy.

Gastrointestinal tract

the gut, from mouth to anus.

Reproductive system

the body parts associated with reproduction.

63. Will I lose my hair?

Many patients undergoing chemotherapy are understandably anxious about hair loss. Your doctor and nurse will discuss the likelihood of this in your case. The likelihood of hair loss and how much to expect depends on the chemotherapy drugs that you receive, how frequently they are given, and the duration of treatment. For many patients, especially women, hair loss can be the most traumatic part of the entire treatment process. Loss of hair is a very obvious change in your appearance and can understandably have a considerable affect on self-esteem. It may be the most visible sign, especially among women, that there is a problem. It can occur in other areas apart from the scalp. A loss of facial hair (mustache and beard), axillary (underarm) hair, and pubic hair occurs with the longer chemotherapy regimens. The hair loss can vary, with some people experiencing thinning and others experiencing complete hair loss. The hair loss associated with chemotherapy usually begins 2 to 4 weeks after your treatment has begun. It is usually temporary and grows back starting 1 to 2 months after the completion of therapy. Your new hair may have a different texture or color; for example, it may grow back curly, whereas before chemotherapy it was straight.

64. How can I cope with hair loss?

First, discuss hair loss with your physician and nurse, your close family members, and/or your friends. You may wish to purchase a wig before your first treatment begins so that the color and texture can be closely matched to your own hair color. Many patients prefer to wear a head scarf or bandana rather than a wig, whereas others prefer no head covering. The best thing to do is whatever feels right to you. The American Cancer Society offers an entire program that addresses hair loss and how it affects your appearance. The program is called "Look Good, Feel Better," and it offers seminars as well as one-on-one appointments with professional hairstylists and makeup artists. They offer fashion tips for wearing scarves as well as wigs. Information about this program is available from the American Cancer Society through a toll-free number (1–800–395-LOOK) that operates 24 hours per day, 7 days per week. The American Cancer Society also offers wigs that are free of charge, and some insurance companies will cover the cost of wigs. Otherwise, the cost should be tax deductible.

65. Will I have nausea and vomiting with treatment?

Years ago patients receiving chemotherapy may have gotten very sick and experienced much vomiting. Today, however, there are many more chemotherapy drugs and other treatments that do not cause significant nausea and/or vomiting. In addition, there are several new antinausea (**antiemetic**) medications that are very effective in preventing this problem. If necessary, your physician will prescribe antinausea drugs along with your chemotherapy. If you are still having nausea or vomiting, inform your doctor or nurse so that they can alter your antinausea drug regimen. Do not assume that you have to tough it out. Also, because everybody responds differently to different regimens, the first antinausea regimen may not work well for you, and alternatives are available. Sometimes a small dose of a steroid can be beneficial when added to other antinausea medications.

Also, rather than eating regular-sized meals, eating several smaller meals throughout the day can be helpful. You should avoid fried or fatty foods and should eat and drink slowly. Although rest is also helpful after a meal, you should not lie flat for at least 2 hours after eating.

66. Do I need to change my diet?

Good nutrition, although frequently neglected in the American diet, is important. The same applies, even more so, as you proceed in your fight against lymphoma. What "good nutrition" means will vary according to your specific circumstances. Consulting with a dietician can be helpful. Eating adequate amounts of a healthy diet can help you feel better in general. When your body is receiving all that it needs, your ability to tolerate the side effects of the lymphoma and its treatment is increased, and you may also decrease your chance of infection through a beneficial effect on the immune system. A healthy diet and good nutrition will enhance your ability to maintain your strength and energy level, counteracting fatigue.

For those of you who do not have any specific problems that interfere with your appetite or ability to eat, we suggest that you follow the Food Guide Pyramid (Figure 5). This is an outline of what to eat daily based on guidelines set by the U.S. Department of Agriculture. Use this as a rough guide, possibly adding one to two servings from the milk group and one to two servings from the meat group. This will increase your total protein intake, which often is needed during an illness.

Changing your diet is a relatively easy step to take and is an aspect of your health in which you can have direct control. This is important at a time when you may feel that so many things fall outside of your control. Making your diet healthier may carry the benefits discussed previously, but as far as we know will not directly treat the lymphoma.

If you have lost weight, you may be able to focus on increasing your protein and energy (caloric) intake. If

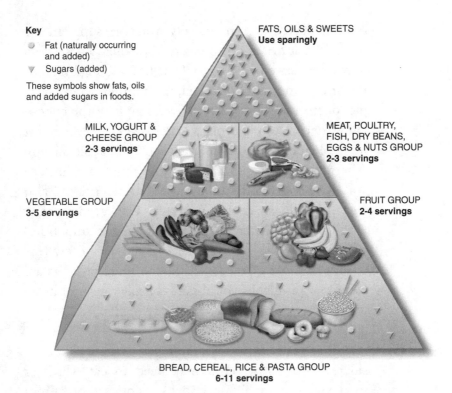

Key

- Fat (naturally occurring and added)
- Sugars (added)

These symbols show fats, oils and added sugars in foods.

FATS, OILS & SWEETS
Use sparingly

MILK, YOGURT &
CHEESE GROUP
2-3 servings

MEAT, POULTRY,
FISH, DRY BEANS,
EGGS & NUTS GROUP
2-3 servings

VEGETABLE GROUP
3-5 servings

FRUIT GROUP
2-4 servings

BREAD, CEREAL, RICE & PASTA GROUP
6-11 servings

Figure 5   The Food Guide Pyramid. Source: USDA.

your appetite is good, this is fairly easy to accomplish. Focus on eating more high-calorie foods that provide protein, such as milk, cheese, and eggs. Sauces and gravies are also an efficient way of obtaining more calories.

If your appetite is poor, the same high-calorie and high-protein diet is encouraged. Try to eat several (five or six) small meals throughout the day and to include high-protein snacks such as ice cream, pudding, cheese, and peanut butter. At those times when you are not able to face a meal, a nourishing drink is an acceptable alternative. You can also add these drinks between meals to help with weight gain.

Several different commercially available supplements can add calories and protein to your diet. These taste best when served very cold. If the taste of one brand or flavor does not appeal to you, try another. Many people "doctor up" these drinks; for example, if the chocolate variety is too chocolaty or too sweet, try mixing it in a blender with some milk or vanilla ice cream. Alternatively, try adding some fruit, milk, or other flavor of ice cream to a vanilla variety drink. You can also create a milk shake from scratch. Or, combine milk with various fruits or fruit yogurt to make a "smoothie." You can also add a scoop of ice cream and a few teaspoons of protein powder. Although these powders are commonly available, you should consult your healthcare team before using any dietary supplements.

At times you may want some foods that may be considered "unhealthy." You may need to eat whatever food you can to obtain enough calories. Sometimes you may need to think of food like medicine: take some every 2 to 3 hours whether you feel like it or not. Be conscious of what you are eating but, on the other hand, do not become obsessed. Mealtimes should be enjoyable and not a source of stress.

If you do not feel like preparing a meal, frozen dinners and microwaveable foods are convenient. This is also a perfect opportunity to give family and friends the chance to help you (e.g., going to the grocery store or doing some cooking). If you have times when your energy level is better and you enjoy cooking, you could prepare some meals in advance and freeze them for later. If you really cannot face preparing or eating a meal, have one of the nutritional supplements discussed previously. Of course, eating out is an alternative. At certain times during chemotherapy, especially when your white blood cell count is low, your may be restricted to a **low microbial diet**—one that limits your exposure to food-borne bacteria or fungi.

Low microbial diet

a diet containing low amounts of bacteria or fungi.

67. What should I do if I'm having side effects that interfere with eating?

A sore throat or mouth sores from chemotherapy or radiation can result in difficulty eating. Crunchy foods such as raw fruits and vegetables, dry breads and cereals, spicy foods, and citrus should be avoided. Instead, eat soft and creamy food such as yogurt, pudding, buttered noodles, and cooked cereal. You may also find that foods that are too hot can also cause discomfort. Lukewarm or cool foods tend to be more soothing.

If you cannot tolerate solids, try liquid foods such as cream soups or nutrition drinks and shakes.

If nausea or vomiting is a problem, try sipping fluids throughout the day (along with trying antinausea medications), because you need to drink enough fluids to prevent **dehydration**. Water is good, but juice-type commercial supplements may be even better. These provide protein as well as calories.

Dehydration

low fluids in the body, which can cause dizziness, fatigue, fainting, and other minor symptoms. If not corrected, dehydration can cause more serious problems.

If you're feeling queasy but are not vomiting, try eating bland foods that are easy to digest (e.g., crackers, toast, rice, gelatin, and sherbet). These foods are not adequate sources of protein, calories, or nutrients, but this diet can be followed for a few days until the nausea subsides, as long as you are drinking enough liquids.

Sometimes food that you have previously enjoyed may taste bland. This can be the result of various medications, including chemotherapy. This change in taste may result in a loss of appetite and a failure to obtain adequate nutrition. Again, treating food like medicine—eating small amounts at regular intervals—may be a way to overcome this problem. You may need to experiment with new foods or new seasonings, or may need to add additional sugar, salt, or other flavor to enhance the taste. Most people report that cold or room-temperature foods are less offensive in their smell and taste.

Anorexia

loss of appetite.

Megestrol acetate

a medication that can increase the appetite.

If you simply have no appetite (**anorexia**), you may benefit from **megestrol acetate** (Megace), which is a hormonal agent that can stimulate the appetite and result in a weight gain. This is an option that you should discuss with your physician.

68. How do I cope with anemia?

Anemia is common in patients with lymphoma. A blood test measures the hemoglobin level, or the **hematocrit**. Symptoms of anemia include fatigue, weakness, shortness of breath, headache, ringing in your ears, **palpitations** (an increased awareness of the heart beating), nausea, and occasional chest pain.

Hematocrit

a measure of the number of red cells, useful for anemia or polycythemia (too many red cells).

Palpitations

the sensation of an irregular heart beat.

Anemia can occur for many different reasons. Often bone marrow reacts to lymphoma in your body by decreasing the production of red blood cells. This also happens in people with many other illnesses, not just cancer. It occurs with infections and arthritis. This type of anemia is called anemia of chronic disease.

Lymphoma involving the bone marrow can also cause anemia. Bleeding can obviously lead to anemia and also needs to be considered as a cause. If bleeding occurs, report it to your physician. Having black tarry bowel movements is a sign of bleeding in the bowels and requires urgent attention.

Chemotherapy commonly causes or worsens anemia and may contribute to fatigue (Question 71). You should note that anemia is only one of many factors that contribute to fatigue.

Your doctor may perform tests to determine the reasons for the anemia. Deficiencies of iron, vitamin B12, or folic acid are possible causes that simple blood tests can easily evaluate. If any of these are deficient, supplements can be provided. More commonly, anemia is not due to any deficiency in your diet and is therefore unlikely to respond to dietary supplements. Question 71 discusses the use of **erythropoietin** in preventing or treating anemia.

When you have symptoms from anemia, you should not overdo activities. Exercising is generally a good thing and should be encouraged but not pushed too hard. Limiting your activities to what you feel up to and getting plenty of rest can help to improve your sense of well-being.

69. Why is having a low white blood count such a concern?

Another common effect of chemotherapy is the reduction of the white blood cell count (**neutropenia**), which increases the risk of developing an infection. Crowds and people with colds or flu should be avoided, but in reality, the most common infections during periods of a low blood count actually arise from within your own body. A neutropenic or low microbial

Erythropoietin

a hormone produced by the kidneys that stimulates the bone marrow to produce red blood cells.

Neutropenia

a low level of neutrophils.

The most common infections during periods of a low blood count actually arise from within your own body.

diet may help to prevent some of these infections. The chance of an infection is increased for older patients or for those with other medical problems such as chronic lung disease or diabetes. Having a central venous catheter also increases the chance of an infection. Even if you take precautions, infections are not entirely preventable. The risk of infection is highest with lower white blood cell counts and is also related to longer durations of neutropenia. Certain chemotherapy drugs or combinations of drugs are associated with a higher risk of infections than others.

If a fever develops while you are receiving chemotherapy or in the period afterward when your white count is low, you should seek medical attention without delay, especially if it is above 100.5°F. With neutropenia, infections can progress very rapidly and can even result in death if antibiotics are not started promptly.

It is a good idea to keep a weekend bag packed.

The development of a fever may result in a hospital admission. For this reason, it is a good idea to keep a weekend bag packed. Sometimes, after being assessed, an outpatient antibiotic treatment may be adequate. First, blood samples should be obtained before starting antibiotics to identify the cause of the infection. You will also have a chest x-ray, and a urine culture will need to be examined.

Depending on the chemotherapy that you receive and on other factors such as your age and general health, your physician may prescribe a white blood cell growth factor in an effort to allow your white blood cell count to recover sooner after chemotherapy. Most commonly, granulocyte-colony stimulating factor, or G-CSF (Neupogen), is used for this purpose. It is administered by a daily subcutaneous injection until the white blood cell count has recovered. A newer, chemically altered version of Neupogen, called Neulasta, has recently become available. It remains in the circulation for a considerably longer period of time until the white blood cell count recovers and therefore only needs to be given once with every chemotherapy cycle. Like Neupogen, Neulasta is given as a subcutaneous injection.

Not everybody on chemotherapy needs to get a white blood cell growth factor. The decision is based on how likely you are to get an infection while on chemotherapy and whether you have previously experienced an infection. Discuss the need for a growth factor with your physician. The American Society of Clinical Oncology has developed guidelines for when these growth factors should be administered.

70. How do lymphoma and its treatment affect my sexuality?

It is not uncommon for lymphoma and its treatment to bring about physical and/or emotional changes that affect your sexual relationship. The degree to which this occurs depends on several factors, including the stage and symptoms of your lymphoma, the treatment that you are undergoing, as well as your overall emotional state.

It is difficult for some people to initiate conversations about sexuality with their partner; however, it can be very beneficial to speak openly and honestly with each other about your needs and wants. If you cannot do this, you might find it helpful to see a counselor or therapist on a short-term basis.

Although it may be even harder to discuss sexuality with strangers, a discussion with your healthcare team may help you to adjust to any changes as they occur. If your doctor or nurse is not helpful, speaking to the social worker may be beneficial.

One common issue that you may face as a result of your lymphoma and your treatment is a decreased sex drive, which can be a direct effect of your treatment or associated with fatigue or stress. It is important that this does not become the cause of further stress in your relationship. With good communication, your partner should understand the reasons for the decreased **libido**. You can also remind your partner that this is a temporary disruption, and once treatment (or the fatigue associated with it) is over, your sex drive will return to its former level. Depression, which is treatable, should also be considered as a possible cause for decreased libido.

Libido

sex drive.

Chemotherapy and radiation can cause dryness of a woman's vagina. A water-soluble lubricant can help ease discomfort associated with decreased vaginal lubrication. Also, keep an open mind that there are different ways to feel sexual pleasure, as there may be times when intercourse is not possible. It is very important that you and your partner continue other ways of expressing affection for each other. Sometimes just cuddling can be enough, or you may want to explore other ways of caressing and stimulating each other. Chemotherapy and radiation can also result in low **testosterone** levels, which result in difficulty obtaining or maintaining an erection. Replacing testosterone may be all that is required. If your white blood cell or platelet count is low (50,000 is usually the minimum requirement), sexual intercourse may not be advisable; you should discuss this with your healthcare team.

Some people choose to wait to focus on the sexual part of their relationship until treatment is complete. Only you and your partner can decide what is best. Honesty and open communication avoid hurt feelings and mis-understandings and are an important part of resuming normal sexual activity.

71. Is fatigue always due to chemotherapy?

Fatigue, a very common symptom for many patients with cancer, can vary from slight fatigue, making every-day activities slightly more burdensome, to profound fatigue, resulting in extreme difficulty even getting out of bed. Fatigue can be extremely incapacitating, result-ing in major impairment in quality of life, and is com-mon even in patients who are not receiving chemotherapy. Many causes of fatigue exist among cancer patients, with anemia being one. This may be related to lymphoma's bone marrow involvement, resulting in decreased red blood cell production. Even without bone marrow involvement, anemia of chronic disease may also be present and may contribute to fatigue, which cytokine production can cause. Cytokines are chemicals that tumor cells produce in response to an infection. Lymphoma patients are understandably under a lot of stress, which is another cause of fatigue. Depression can add to the fatigue. Medications should also be evaluated as an additional factor that contributes to stress.

Discuss fatigue with your physician or nurse if it is an issue.

Discuss fatigue with your physician or nurse if it is an issue. If anemia is a significant component causing fatigue, a blood transfusion may be necessary. Erythropoietin is available for injection and may be beneficial in some circumstances (the kidneys produce erythropoietin, which then travels to the bone marrow cells and stimulates the production of red blood cells). It is available as a medication in a number of different preparations. Epoetin alpha (Procrit), which is given by a subcutaneous or intravenous injection, has been used for many years and is very similar to the naturally produced erythropoietin that the kidneys produce. It can be given either three times per week or once per week. A more recently available and longer-acting version, darbopoietin alpha (Aranesp), can be given every two weeks and appears to be similarly effective. Because there are many other causes of fatigue besides anemia, erythropoietin will not benefit all patients. Discuss this with your physician. Your list of medications should also be evaluated. If any medications can be discontinued, this may be helpful. Again, discuss this with your physician.

Maintaining a good caloric intake and adequate hydration is also important in counteracting fatigue. Plan your daily activities with an emphasis on the activities that are more important. It is quite acceptable to take naps, but sleeping too much during the day can further disrupt your sleeping pattern. Some daily exercise as tolerated can also be helpful in managing your fatigue.

72. Does chemotherapy cause bleeding?

Chemotherapy may cause bleeding, which is due to a fall in the platelet count. Regular blood counts are important while you are receiving chemotherapy and will help to detect the need for platelet transfusions. If you develop any abnormal bleeding while on chemotherapy, inform your doctor. Abnormal bruising in addition to bleeding is also important. Other signs of a low platelet count include **petechiae**, which are small, purple, reddish spots on your skin that are actually tiny bleeds. They are most frequently seen on the front of your shins. During periods when your platelet count is low, you should avoid razorblades for shaving (use electric razors instead), nail clippers, and dental floss. For mouth care, you should use only a very soft toothbrush or sponges.

Petechiae

pinpoint red spots that occur with low platelet counts and are due to tiny areas of bleeding in the skin.

The occurrence of low platelet counts during chemotherapy depends on a number of factors, including the type of chemotherapy being administered, the amount of chemotherapy that the patient has previously received, and whether and to what degree the bone marrow is involved with lymphoma. It is important to control high blood pressure when the platelet count is low, as the risk of bleeding may be increased.

Activities such as contact sports that could result in trauma need to be curtailed while the platelet count is low. Discuss any such activities with your physician before participation.

73. What is radiation therapy?

Radiation therapy uses high-energy x-rays to kill or prevent cancer cells from growing. Cancer cells grow faster than normal cells, so they are more susceptible to radiation. Because radiation therapy can also damage normal tissues around the area being radiated, your radiation doctor will try to ensure that only the cancer cells receive the radiation. Before starting radiation treatment, a simulation will be performed, at which time tiny tattoo marks or dots will be placed on your skin to mark the area to be radiated. Areas that are not to receive radiation will be protected with lead shielding. The radiation treatment itself takes only a few minutes, but treatment is spread over a few days to a few weeks, depending on the total dose of radiation to be administered. For treatment, you will generally be lying on a table close to a noisy radiation machine.

Before starting radiation treatment, you will have an appointment with a radiation oncologist, who specializes in radiation therapy to treat cancer. At the initial visit, your case will be reviewed to ensure that you are to benefit from radiation treatment and that the treatment can be given safely. The radiation oncologist will also review any scans or x-ray tests, as these will be helpful for planning the exact area that needs radiation. After this visit, you should have a good understanding of the reasons for needing radiation treatment, what to expect from the radiation in terms of side effects, and how long the treatment course will be.

Radiation is referred to as local treatment, being useful when treating particular sites within the body. The field of treatment is called a radiation port. **Total body irradiation** refers to the radiation of the whole body and is sometimes used in preparation for a transplant.

Total body irradiation

radiation therapy administered to the entire body, usually in preparation for a transplant.

74. Will I need radiation therapy?

Radiation therapy can be useful for the treatment of lymphoma under many different circumstances. It can be used as the only treatment for some patients with stage 1 or stage 2 Hodgkin's disease or indolent lymphoma. In these cases, especially in Hodgkin's disease, it is very important to be certain that the lymphoma is in only these areas. Therefore, accurate staging is very important for planning the correct treatment.

For patients with aggressive non-Hodgkin's lymphoma, radiation, if needed, is usually combined with chemotherapy. In fact, in certain situations, using radiation therapy allows the number of chemotherapy cycles necessary to be reduced, therefore reducing the risk of side effects from chemotherapy exposure. In other situations, the radiation may be an additional treatment aimed at areas where the lymphoma was particularly bulky, in an attempt to reduce the likelihood of recurrence.

Radiation can rapidly control lymphoma at specific sites if necessary. An example of such a need is pain control due to lymphoma growing at one site or lymphoma pressing on the spinal cord causing nerve damage. Spinal cord compression is a very urgent situation in which the lymphoma presses on the spinal cord causing weakness, often in the legs, numbness, and possible loss of control of bladder or bowel function. These symptoms require extremely urgent medical attention, because unless they are corrected rapidly, the nerve damage may be permanent.

75. What are the side effects of radiation therapy?

Radiation therapy itself is painless and does not cause you to become radioactive; however, you may experience some side effects depending on the part of your body that is being radiated. Other factors include the dose of radiation and whether chemotherapy is given at the same time. Side effects may be localized to the body part being treated or can be more widespread. Be sure to report any and all side effects to your healthcare team, as most can be effectively managed. Also remember that although side effects can be unpleasant, most are temporary and will gradually disappear after the treatment is finished.

Be sure to report any and all side effects to your health-care team.

During radiation therapy, the skin in the area being treated may become dry, irritated, and sensitive; it may feel and look sunburned and may also become itchy and then peel. To avoid further irritation, radiated areas should be kept clean using only warm water and very mild cleansers. Your healthcare team may prescribe or recommend creams, lotions, or ointments. You should avoid all cosmetics, deodorants, perfumes, powders, and other products that increase irritation in the affected area and that your healthcare team has not approved. It is also important to avoid sun exposure for a long time after therapy has been completed.

Fatigue, or generalized weakness, is another common side effect of radiation therapy. It tends to increase gradually and is cumulative as radiation continues. By completion of a course of radiation therapy, many patients have a significant degree of fatigue.

Medical problems—including infection, anemia, and dehydration, all of which are treatable—can compound fatigue that is caused by radiation. Your physician should look for any of these aggravating factors. Ways of coping with fatigue include ensuring adequate sleep at night, resting during the day, eating a balanced diet with adequate calories and protein, and exercising at a tolerable level. Light exercise, such as walking and stretching, is helpful. A consultation with a physical therapist may prove helpful for advice on incorporating light exercise into your daily routine.

Radiation can cause a loss of appetite (anorexia) or nausea (Question 65). Radiation treatments to the neck or chest may result in a sore throat or dry mouth, resulting in a condition called **xerostomia**, which results from damage to the salivary glands. Saliva is essential for chewing and swallowing food and is the primary lubricant for food. Inflammation to the **esophagus** (the tube that connects the throat to your stomach) may also occur. This condition, called **esophagitis**, results in painful or difficult swallowing and possibly also heartburn.

If you experience esophagitis or xerostomia, consider eating softer foods or commercially available dietary shakes. You should avoid citrus fruits and juices, as these can be especially irritating. Commercially available saliva substitutes may also be helpful for coping with a dry mouth; your healthcare team can help with this.

Radiation may also cause hair loss to the specific body part being treated. Although this is generally temporary, higher doses can also cause permanency. Unlike chemotherapy, radiation treatment does not cause generalized hair loss.

Xerostomia
dryness of the mouth due to disease.

Esophagus
the tube connecting the throat to the stomach.

Esophagitis
inflammation of the esophagus.

PART SIX

Other Therapies

What is immunotherapy?

What are monoclonal antibodies?

How is rituximab (Rituxan) administered?

More ...

76. What is immunotherapy?

Immunotherapy implies the use of immune molecules or the patient's own immune system to treat the disease. When used to discuss lymphoma, this generally refers to the use of monoclonal antibodies; however, therapeutic vaccines and allogeneic stem cell transplants are also forms of immunotherapy.

77. What are monoclonal antibodies?

Monoclonal antibodies are immunoglobulin proteins that are produced by one population of cells or clone (hence monoclonal). Every antibody is built in the shape of the letter Y. This structure allows the antibody to be useful for fighting infection. It also makes it useful for treating some types of cancer. The arms of the Y have a particular protein sequence that can recognize and attach to small, specific protein targets, termed antigens. The foot of the Y can link to other cells in the immune system that can rid the body of the antigen. Antibodies are vital to a normal immune system, providing essential protection against otherwise potentially fatal infections.

CD20 is an antigen that is present on the lymphoma cells of most patients who have indolent non-Hodgkin's lymphoma. Rituximab (the first immunotherapy that the Food and Drug Administration approved for use in cancer) is an antibody that is designed so that the arms of the Y attach to CD20. When rituximab is infused into the circulation, it seeks out the CD20 that is present on lymphocytes and targets them for destruction.

Recently, a second monoclonal antibody called ibritumomab tiuxetan (Zevalin), also approved for the treatment of indolent lymphoma, also targets CD20 but carries a payload in the form of a radioactive molecule called Ytrium. In this way, radiation is specifically delivered to the lymphoma cells, resulting in less damage to normal body cells. Other monoclonal antibodies are now available for patients with breast cancer and colon cancer, and many more are in clinical trials.

78. How is rituximab (Rituxan) administered?

Rituxan is usually infused intravenously every week for 4 weeks (in some circumstances, for 8 weeks). If given along with chemotherapy, the schedule depends on the chemotherapy regimen. The first time rituxan is infused, patients are likely to experience fever and chills, which can be quite uncomfortable, but this resolves by slowing the infusion. Because of this, the first infusion takes the longest, maybe even 8 hours or more. Subsequent infusions can generally be completed in 4 to 6 hours. Fever and chills occur less often with the remaining infusions. Tylenol and Benadryl can help to reduce the severity of the fever and chills.

79. How is ibritumomab tiuxetan (Zevalin) administered?

Zevalin is more complicated to administer than Rituxan. Because it is a form of radiation treatment (Ytrium), a **nuclear medicine** physician or a radiation oncologist is required for its administration. Only one course of treatment is necessary, but it takes 7 to 9 days. The first administration of Rituxan on day 1 takes a number of hours. Next, a modified form of Zevalin (containing Indium rather than Ytrium) is administered over 10 minutes. It is given to determine

Other Therapies

Nuclear medicine
the medicine specialty that involves using radioisotopes for obtaining body scans and for treatment.

the amount of radiation that different parts of the body will receive when Zevalin is administered. Because of the need for special handling of radiation treatments, it may be necessary to receive the two treatments in different locations, which can be inconvenient.

Within 1 or 2 days, a scan is performed with a **gamma camera** in order to determine the distribution of the radiation in the body. Additional scans may be necessary 2 to 4 days later, depending on the results of the first scan. On days 7 to 9 of treatment, a second dose of Rituxan is given, which is followed by the actual treatment dose of Zevalin. This again may need to be given at a different location. Zevalin itself only takes 10 minutes to infuse.

It is currently recommended that Zevalin be given only to patients whose platelet count is at least 100,000. Zevalin may result in a further drop in blood counts, sometimes resulting in the need for transfusions. A bone marrow examination is also recommended before Zevalin treatment. If more than 25% of the marrow space is involved with lymphoma, Zevalin should not be given, as there is a risk that too much radiation will be concentrated in the marrow, possibly resulting in permanent marrow damage.

80. What are lymphoma vaccines?

You are familiar with vaccines given during childhood to prevent infections. A vaccine is a preparation of a protein given to stimulate an immune response against a particular infection. Vaccination for cancer is a newer concept. In lymphoma, vaccination is experimental, and, currently, patients can receive this treatment only in the setting of a clinical trial.

The aim of treatment is to eliminate lymphoma or to prevent its reoccurrence. With immunization against infectious disease, the aim is to prevent the infection from occurring in the first place.

For a vaccine to be effective in cancer, a protein unique to the cancer cell is needed to stimulate an immune response. For most cancers, this is not currently available, because their proteins also occur on normal cells.

In B-cell lymphomas, the abnormal cells have a single type of immunoglobulin on their surface. This immunoglobulin is an antibody molecule, and part of it is called an **idiotype**. The idiotype is the same for all the lymphoma cells belonging to that patient but differs from the idiotype on other normal lymphocytes and also from the lymphoma of other patients. As a result, the idiotype is an excellent target for vaccination.

Idiotype

a protein sequence on the surface of B lymphocytes that is like a fingerprint. All related lymphocytes contain the same protein sequence.

The first step in producing a lymphoma vaccine is the surgical removal of a lymph node. The specific idiotype is then produced during a process that takes 8 to 16 weeks. Once produced, the idiotype is joined to another large foreign carrier protein that enhances the immune response, and the carrier protein is then ready for injection into the patient. The vaccination is given along with a growth factor, usually GM-CSF (Leukine). The vaccination schedule varies according to the particular clinical trial. To date, a number of clinical centers are conducting clinical trials to determine the best vaccination approach. Thus far, results

Other Therapies

appear promising, and much more information should become available in the near future.

81. What is a bone marrow or stem cell transplant?

A bone marrow or stem cell transplant is a treatment that allows for the administration of higher doses of chemotherapy or radiation than you could receive without the transplant. Currently, the effects on the bone marrow limit the ability to increase the dose of many drugs that are used to treat lymphoma. Being able to increase the dose of the drugs can reduce the chance that the lymphoma will return. In the case of some chemotherapy drugs, this increased dose could destroy the bone marrow. If such a case were to occur, a very high risk of infection is likely, and patients would require regular transfusions of both red blood cells and platelets. In order to avoid this complication, a bone marrow or stem cell transplant can be performed.

A bone marrow transplant, as the name suggests, involves actually using the bone marrow cells for the transplant. Obtaining the bone marrow requires an operation with a general anesthetic. In the past 10 years, most transplant centers obtain bone marrow stem cells from the blood circulation rather than directly from the bone marrow. Such transplants are called **peripheral blood stem cell transplants**. Although obtained from the blood, the stem cells are still bone marrow stem cells, but they move into the bloodstream after treatment with growth factors such as G-CSF (Neupogen). Stem cells also move into the blood circulation as blood counts recover after chemotherapy. Often a patient's own stem cells are

Peripheral blood stem cell transplants

a transplant using marrow stem cells that have been obtained from the blood circulation.

collected after the administration of both chemotherapy and white blood cell growth factors. When transplanted back into the patient after high-dose chemotherapy, the stem cells are able to produce red cells, white cells, and platelets. Using marrow stem cells obtained from the blood as opposed to the marrow results in a significantly shorter period of low blood counts. This has made these types of transplant considerably safer.

82. Why is a transplant used for treating lymphoma?

Basically, there are two main mechanisms by which a transplant can be useful in treating lymphoma. First, it enables the safer delivery of much higher doses of chemotherapy than would otherwise be possible. The higher doses of chemotherapy may cure an aggressive lymphoma or prevent an indolent lymphoma from returning for a longer period of time than after regular doses of chemotherapy. An **allogeneic transplant** (somebody else's bone marrow cells) offers the additional advantage of providing normal bone marrow cells from a healthy donor. Therefore, there is no chance of lymphoma cells being returned with the transplant. Second, in the case of an allogeneic transplant, an additional and important benefit is the introduction of the donor's immune system. In some types of lymphoma, the donors' immune system can then recognize your lymphoma cells as foreign and destroy them. In this way, an allogeneic transplant is a potential cure for some types of indolent lymphoma and Hodgkin's disease. This effect is called **graft versus lymphoma** (GVL). Unfortunately, similar types of immune cells from the healthy donor that cause GVL

Other Therapies

Graft versus lymphoma

a situation in which the donor's immune system recognizes the recipient's lymphoma cells as foreign and works to eliminate the lymphoma.

can cause graft-versus-host disease (GVHD). In this condition, the donor's immune cells recognize the patient's body as foreign, attacking certain organs and body parts. GVHD can often be treated and controlled but sometimes can cause a more serious problem or even death. The chance that GVHD will occur and perhaps be more difficult to control rises significantly for older patients. This and other transplant-related problems are reasons why an allogeneic transplant is not often considered a good choice for older patients. GVHD and GVL occur only with an allogeneic transplant. An autologous transplant does not have the benefit of GVL. It therefore relies on the high doses of chemotherapy to cure lymphoma. Because of the immune benefit of GVL, allogeneic transplants do not necessarily need high doses of chemotherapy. Over the past few years, the concept of a **mini-transplant** or **nonmyeloablative stem cell transplant** has been introduced as possibly a safer method of performing allogeneic transplants. In this way, the benefit of GVL is becoming increasingly available to older patients who previously would have not been eligible for a regular allogeneic transplant (Question 86) (Table 11).

Mini-transplant

a transplant in which the doses of chemotherapy or radiotherapy are reduced compared to those given for a standard transplant.

Nonmyeloablative stem cell transplant

same as mini-transplant.

83. What is an autologous transplant?

An autologous transplant uses your own bone marrow or blood stem cells to restore the blood counts after high-dose chemotherapy. It is used to treat lymphoma in certain situations in which the lymphoma is likely to respond to much higher doses of chemotherapy than can be given without the transplant. The higher doses of chemotherapy can also destroy the bone marrow. Therefore, before giving the high-dose therapy, stem cells are collected from the patient and are frozen.

Table 11 Different types of bone marrow or blood stem cell transplants

Transplant Type	Source of Stem Cells	Preparative Regimen
Autologous	Stem cells obtained from the patient's own blood or bone marrow	High-dose therapy
Allogeneic 　Sibling 　Unrelated donor 　Cord blood transplant	Matched stem cells from a 　Sibling 　Volunteer donor 　Umbilical cord blood stem cell 　bank	High-dose therapy
Miniallogeneic (nonmyeloablative)	Sibling or unrelated donor	Reduced-dose therapy

Other Therapies

After the high-dose chemotherapy, the stem cells are thawed and infused back into the patient. After a period of usually 1.5 to 2 weeks, the stem cells start making all of the different types of blood cells. The cells that recover most rapidly are the white blood cells. The number of stem cells obtained before the transplant affects how fast the stem cells recover. Faster recovery occurs with higher numbers of stem cells. For appropriate patients, the risks of an autologous transplant are low. Because the blood counts drop after the high-dose chemotherapy, there is a higher risk of infection. If this occurs, intravenous antibiotics are required. Platelet transfusions are often needed to reduce the risk of bleeding, and blood transfusions are often required to manage anemia.

Many transplant centers perform autologous transplants as an outpatient. When performed as an outpatient, it is important that you have someone available at home to help and to drive you to the hospital for the frequent visits (often daily) that are required. If any complication such as a fever, occurs, you would be admitted to the hospital.

84. How is an autologous transplant performed?

The procedure for an autologous transplant involves a number of steps. If your lymphoma specialist recommends an autologous transplant, a number of tests are necessary to try to ensure that you are well enough to tolerate the high-dose therapy and the following period of low blood counts. These tests include evaluations of your heart, lung, and kidney function in addition to an assessment of your general well-being. Blood tests to detect any infections, such as hepatitis, will also be obtained. Approval from your insurance company is also required. Next, a **pheresis catheter**, which is usually placed in the upper chest wall, is necessary for collecting stem cells from your blood. **Stem cell mobilization** is the next step, whereby the bone marrow stem cells are stimulated to move into the blood circulation. For stem cell mobilization, white blood cell growth factors given alone or with chemotherapy are administered. The stem cell collection will then be scheduled as the white blood cell count recovers. The collection of the stem cells involves a procedure called **leukapheresis**, for which you are connected to a leukapheresis machine via your pheresis catheter. A small amount of your blood volume is transferred into the machine where the white blood cells are separated from the red blood cells and the platelets. The white cells contain the bone marrow stem cells and are collected in a special bag to be frozen. The red cells and platelets are returned to your circulation. The leukapheresis often needs to be

Pheresis catheter

a large indwelling catheter placed through the skin into a large vein to allow the collection of stem cells.

Stem cell mobilization

the process by which bone marrow stem cells are stimulated to move into the blood circulation.

Leukapheresis

a procedure to remove large numbers of white blood cells from the body.

repeated over a few days in order to get an adequate number of stem cells. The procedure on the machine takes approximately 4 to 6 hours.

The stem cells are then frozen along with a chemical protectant called DMSO, which is responsible for the strange garlic-like taste and smell that you may notice when your stem cells are returned to your body. The next stage of the transplant involves managing the side effects of the high-dose chemotherapy and awaiting the recovery of the blood counts. The transplant team will discuss common side effects of the high-dose chemotherapy with you.

85. What are the complications of an autologous transplant?

Problems can relate to having a pheresis catheter, the leukapheresis procedure, the high doses of chemotherapy, and the resulting low blood counts before bone marrow recovery.

Problems related to the pheresis catheter. These complications are similar to those that can occur with the placement of a central venous catheter, as discussed in Question 61.

Problems related to leukapheresis. Leukapheresis is generally a painless procedure (unless you consider boredom to be painful). The leukapheresis machine removes a small amount of your blood volume at a time, separating the bone marrow stem cells from the other blood cells. Patients are closely monitored to ensure that too much blood is not removed at any one time. Sometimes dizziness (lightheadedness or a feeling of faintness) may occur. If so, the machine settings can be adjusted or a little extra fluid can be given to adjust for the blood volume that is outside of the body at any time. In addition, because the blood outside of the body cannot be allowed to clot, an anticoagulant is added to your blood that can bind calcium. This can result in a fall in the blood calcium that may result in tingling in the fingers and face. Again, adjustments can be made to the machine settings to compensate for these abnormalities, or you may be given extra calcium (such as Tums). Therefore, it is important to inform your nurse if you are experiencing any discomfort. If you have a low platelet count before leukapheresis, the procedure can result in a farther fall, and you may need a platelet transfusion before the procedure.

Problems related to chemotherapy. The high-dose chemotherapy may cause nausea and vomiting, which can be prevented with good antinausea drugs; thus, severe nausea is much less common these days. Hair loss is very common, usually occurring after about a week. When this begins, you may prefer to shave your head, as the continuing hair loss can be quite messy. Chemotherapy can damage the lining of the gut. The mouth, all of the way through to the anus, can be affected, resulting in mouth pain, chest pain similar to heartburn, abdominal pain, diarrhea, and rectal pain. Different chemotherapy regimens cause this to varying degrees. Medication can keep you comfortable if the pain becomes unpleasant. A regimen of mouth care that is designed to maintain high levels of oral hygiene will be started with the high-dose chemotherapy. Frequent mouth cleaning with sponges and a mouthwash will lessen the chance of complications, although it may not prevent breakdown. The high doses of chemotherapy can occasionally have damaging effects on other normal body parts. The degree to which this happens depends on the exact type of drug used, and your transplant team will discuss this with you. Possible effects, which are unusual, include damage to the lungs, heart, liver, bladder, or kidneys. During the time that chemotherapy is given and in the days afterward, your will be examined daily to assess for any evidence of organ damage from the chemotherapy. Blood tests are also obtained for the same reason. Rare complications can arise even after you appear to have completely recovered from the transplant and have returned home. One such side effect relates to the very active drug BCNU, which is for treating lymphoma and is commonly used in the high-dose therapy regimens. It can cause an inflammation in the lungs, referred to as **BCNU pneumonitis**, which can result in a cough, a shortness of breath, or a fever developing even up to a year after the transplant. It can be effectively treated with a course of steroids. Therefore, if these symptoms develop, you should contact your physician without delay.

GVHD does not occur after an autologous transplant. Immune-suppressing medications are therefore not required. Patients do not normally need to be on steroids after an autologous transplantation.

Problems related to low blood counts. These are discussed in Question 69.

86. What is an allogeneic transplant?

An allogeneic transplant uses bone marrow stem cells of a normal donor. The donor (preferably siblings or occasionally anonymous donors) generally needs to be

Other Therapies

BCNU pneumonitis
inflammation of the lungs caused by the chemotherapy drug BCNU.

compatible in terms of a number of genetic similarities. To ensure this, special testing referred to as **human leukocyte antigen (HLA) typing** is performed on both the patient and potential donors.

Human leukocyte antigen typing

testing of the transplantation antigens to determine whether two people are compatible for transplantation.

The HLA system consists of a set of different proteins present on most cells in the body. Six of these proteins are very important for the purposes of a transplant and are transmitted from your parents in two groups of three proteins each. The three proteins in each group are usually passed on together. Each parent provides one set of the proteins to each child. As one of the sets comes from each parent, there is a 25% chance that each brother and sister, as long as they share the same parents, will have the same set of proteins and therefore will have identical HLA. It is rare for other relatives besides brothers or sisters to be HLA identical as they do not share parents and, therefore, have inherited different HLA proteins. In rare situations, however, it is worthwhile to test children or parents.

If there are no matched siblings, an allogeneic transplant may still be possible, but an unrelated donor would then need to be found. A transplant using an HLA-identical donor other than a sibling is referred to as a matched unrelated donor transplant. An organization, the National Marrow Donor Program, maintains a registry of millions of HLA-typed volunteers who are prepared to donate marrow stem cells. For HLA typing, a blood sample is obtained, and a bone marrow evaluation is unnecessary. If you are a possible candidate for an unrelated donor transplant, you can be referred to a transplant center where a search of the registry can be initiated.

The side effects and risks of an allogeneic transplant are quite different from those of an autologous transplant. The fundamental reason is that, along with the new bone marrow cells, you acquire the immune system of your donor. This can be beneficial due to the GVL effect whereby the new immune cells recognize lymphoma cells as foreign and act to eliminate them. This can result in treatment benefits that are unavailable using only chemotherapy. The downside is GVHD (discussed in Question 88).

87. How is an allogeneic transplant performed?

An allogeneic transplant differs from an autologous transplant in a number of ways. Two people are involved—you and your donor. For matched unrelated donor transplants, the National Marrow Donor Program arranges the collection or harvesting of the bone marrow stem cells. These are obtained either directly from the bone marrow during a surgical procedure with general anesthesia or from the blood circulation using leukapheresis. If leukapheresis is performed, as discussed in Question 84, the donor receives a white blood cell growth factor to stimulate stem cells into the blood. Once the stem cells are obtained, they are shipped to the transplant center for infusion into the patient. Before stem cell collection, a physician evaluates and screens the donor for any illness or infectious disease that would make it unsafe. In cases in which the donor is a family member, your transplant physician will arrange for stem cell collection. Once obtained, the stem cells either can be frozen or infused directly into the transplant recipient. Whether they are fresh or frozen, there is no difference in outcome to the recipient. The therapy given to you just before you receive the transplant is designed, except in the case of the minitransplant, to eliminate any remaining lymphoma. It is also designed to eliminate your bone marrow and immune system to ensure that your immune system does not reject the new bone marrow cells. The high-dose therapy may consist of chemotherapy alone or may be combined with radiation therapy to the whole body (called total body irradiation). You will generally be hospitalized for these treatments, although in some centers the radiation may be arranged as an outpatient treatment, usually twice a day over 3 days.

Medications will be provided to prevent nausea and vomiting. After the chemotherapy, a rest day is usual to allow for elimination of drugs from the body. The new bone marrow stem cells are then infused into your bloodstream through a catheter. The day that you receive the new stem cells is referred to as day 0. Then the waiting period for the new cells to start producing all of the blood cells begins. During this period your blood counts will be low, and the risks for an infection are highest. You will likely also need platelet and red cell transfusions. The chemotherapy or total body irradiation often results in **mucositis** (a breakdown in the lining of the gut), which can last for a number of days. Morphine may be required for adequate pain control.

Mucositis

a painful condition due to breakdown of the lining of the mouth.

Your transplant team will observe you closely to guard against and manage any complications that may arise. After a period of 10 to 14 days, but sometimes as long as 3 weeks, the new stem cells begin to produce blood cells. The white blood count is usually the first of the blood types to recover, often rising to a normal level over a period of only a few days. It is during the time of white cell recovery and the following weeks that GVHD is most likely to occur. The platelet count recovers more slowly than the white count.

88. What is graft–versus–host disease?

Graft-versus-host disease or GVHD is the syndrome in which lymphocytes derived from the donor can recognize the recipient's body as foreign. The donor lymphocytes essentially attempt to reject the recipient's body. In a kidney or liver transplant patient with a normal immune system, antirejection drugs are given to prevent the patient from rejecting the new kidney or liver. In the case of a bone marrow recipient, their immune system has been eliminated, and thus, the new transplanted immune system attempts to reject the recipient. GVHD can be either acute or chronic. Acute GVHD tends to occur when white cells first appear or in the weeks after the transplant. Characteristically, it affects the skin, liver, and/or the gut. It can cause a skin rash that can be affect any area, but in milder cases it may affect only the palms and soles as well as the ear lobes. When the gut is affected, diarrhea occurs. Blood tests or the presence of jaundice detects liver involvement.

Medication, called cyclosporine A or a related drug called FK506 (Tacrolimus), is given to prevent GVHD. Another drug called methotrexate, a chemotherapy drug, is also useful in low doses after the transplant to prevent GVHD.

Acute GVHD is scored from 1 to 4 according to the severity of the rash, diarrhea, and the abnormal liver tests. If it is grade 1, your transplant physician may

Other Therapies

choose not to treat it, because some degree of GVHD can be beneficial, as GVL may accompany the GVHD. In cases in which the GVHD is more severe, treatment is needed.

The first treatment for GVHD is usually a steroid, which is given orally or intravenously. The medicines used in the attempt to prevent GVHD are also continued. Other medications will be added if the steroids fail to control the GVHD.

Chronic GVHD may occur at any time after the transplant. It may follow directly from acute GVHD or arise without the occurrence of acute GVHD. Chronic GVHD affects individuals differently than acute GVHD. It may result in dry eyes or a dry mouth. It can affect the skin, resulting in skin thickening. If severe, this can affect the joints, resulting in stiffening. The treatment of chronic GVHD is similar to acute GVHD, but there is increasing evidence that Thalidomide can be beneficial.

89. What are mini-transplants?

The rationale for this type of transplant is discussed in Question 82. Essentially, it is a modification of the traditional allogeneic transplant designed to allow the benefits of GVL to be offered to more patients, including older individuals. The lower dose of chemotherapy or radiation given before receiving the donor stem cells is intended to prevent rejection of the new cells, not to eliminate lymphoma. The idea is that the new immune system will work to eliminate the lymphoma. This takes time, and therefore this type of transplant is not felt to be suitable for patients with rapidly growing lymphoma. Also, the best GVL effect is seen among patients with indolent lymphoma. It appears likely that the complication rate for this sort of transplant is lower, partly because it has less affect on normal body tissues from the lower doses of chemotherapy. Tissue damage contributes to GVHD by releasing cytokines. In the minitransplant setting, this is minimized with, hopefully, less GVHD while still allowing GVL to occur. One major research goal in transplant is to separate the cells causing GVHD from those that can cause GVL. Currently, this goal remains elusive.

90. When should I have a transplant?

This is a complicated issue and depends on your type of lymphoma, your response to previous treatment, your age, and your overall general condition. The answer is therefore addressed depending on lymphoma type.

Indolent Lymphoma

Because indolent lymphoma tends to occur in older individuals, most patients are not candidates for an allogeneic transplant. A minitransplant can be considered in certain circumstances. A HLA-matching sibling is usually required, but sometimes a matched unrelated donor may be acceptable. The treatment is currently considered experimental, but some studies suggest that this type of transplant may actually cure some patients. The possibility of a cure results from the "GVL" effect. This treatment option should be considered, especially in younger patients with a suitable donor.

An autologous transplant is an option for a greater number of patients. It does not provide a cure, but in many instances it can provide an extended period before the lymphoma returns. Because autologous transplants have a low risk of serious complications, they are frequently considered. Extending the time before another course of treatment is needed may be a significant advantage for many patients.

Many clinical studies are being conducted in an attempt to improve the results of autologous transplants. Such studies include attempts to purge the bone marrow stem cells before the transplant. **Purging** refers to the removal of any lymphoma cells that may contaminate the stem cells. Methods of purging include treating the stem cells in the laboratory with chemotherapy or antibodies targeting lymphoma cells. This is called ex vivo purging. Treating the patient with chemotherapy or antibodies before collecting the stem cells is a method of in vivo purging. It is not yet clear whether purging results in a better outcome. Ongoing studies are addressing prevention of lymphoma recurrence after an autologous transplant. Such approaches include the use of antibody treatments such as Rituxan or vaccination strategies.

Purging
the technique whereby certain cells (usually cancerous) are removed from the remaining cells present in the collected bone marrow or stem cells.

Aggressive Lymphoma

The aggressive lymphomas include the intermediate- and high-grade lymphomas. The GVL effect that can cure some indolent lymphomas appears to be less effective for these lymphomas. Therefore, an allogeneic transplant is performed less frequently for these disorders. However, for many patients whose lymphoma returns after the initial CHOP (with or without Rituximab), an autologous transplant is often the next recommended treatment (Question 83). Remember, these lymphomas can still be cured with a transplant. As previously noted, patients whose lymphoma continues to respond to regular doses of chemotherapy are the best candidates for transplantation. There may also be patients who at the time their lymphoma is first diagnosed appear to be at a particularly high risk of the lymphoma recurring after chemotherapy. The IPI can help to identify such patients. Currently, clinical studies are ongoing, attempting to determine whether performing an autologous transplant immediately after completing the first course of chemotherapy can prevent the lymphoma from recurring, thereby increasing the cure rate.

Patients whose lymphoma continues to respond to regular doses of chemotherapy are the best candidates for transplantation.

Hodgkin's Disease

Hodgkin's disease is curable in a significant number of patients with radiation therapy, chemotherapy, or a combination of both. If the lymphoma recurs after you have received only radiation, chemotherapy alone may cure the disease. If the recurrence follows chemotherapy, especially if it returns within a short period after completing the therapy, a transplant may be necessary. Most often, an autologous transplant is recommended, but in some situations an allogeneic transplant will be recommended.

91. Should I seek complementary therapy?

Conventional therapies, including such treatments as chemotherapy, monoclonal antibody therapy, and radiation therapy, are treatments that medical doctors recommend. These treatments have been demonstrated in clinical trials to provide the most anticancer activity. Obviously, these treatments are far from perfect, and much work remains to be done. Because of the failings of conventional treatments, interest in **complementary therapy** and **alternative therapy** is high.

Complementary therapy

therapies used in conjunction with traditional medical treatments.

Alternative therapy

a therapy other than a conventionally accepted medical treatment.

Complementary therapies are techniques or approaches that are used in addition to standard or conventional treatments. Examples include meditation, acupuncture, relaxation and massage, visualization, and diet and herbal regimens. Many of these treatments are derived from traditional healing practices and can be important additions to the more traditional treatments. They often help individuals to cope better and feel more in control. Oncologists recognize many complementary therapies for their positive effects on a patient's sense of well-being. The medical community accepts and encourages therapies such as relaxation and visualization. In many cancer centers, you can receive instruction and learn the techniques of various complementary therapies. It is advisable to discuss these therapies with your physician. Rarely, there may be specific reasons why you should avoid a specific complementary therapy.

Meditation and relaxation have been demonstrated to help obtain relief from nausea, anxiety, depression, and stress. Many ways exist to practice meditation and relaxation, and many books and tapes are available at libraries and bookstores. You may need to experiment with a few different techniques before you find one that works for you.

The positive effects of such complementary techniques on the outcome of lymphoma are unknown. Although there is no concrete evidence that such techniques can directly influence lymphoma, indirect effects may exist via subtle changes in the immune system. No harm is brought from such interventions, especially if they help patients to feel more in control.

92. Should I seek alternative therapy?

Alternative therapy, in contrast to complementary therapy, is the substitution of standard medical treatments with unproven and unconventional treatments. In many cases, even lymphoma that has recurred may be curable, so it is heartbreaking to see vulnerable patients decline such potentially curable therapy for alternative remedies without proven benefit. The use of such therapies may result in the loss of an opportunity for a cure.

Lymphoma patients, like all cancer patients, are vulnerable and may be disillusioned with their physician or medical clinic or feel bitter as a result of a relapse. In these situations, it is natural to reach out toward any hope.

Many claims are made for many different remedies. Often, the actual nature of the remedy is not disclosed, and such treatments may cost large sums of money. Usually little or no evidence supports the use of the remedy apart from a list of testimonials from "cured patients."

We would simply advise caution. You expect your lymphoma specialist to have a good rationale for the treatments that he or she prescribes. Hold alternative therapy practitioners to the same standard. Often, alternative therapy practitioners will state that only large pharmaceutical companies can afford to conduct such research. It has been suggested that these same companies even obstruct alternative therapy practitioners from conducting such research. Whatever the reason for the lack of studies and evidence regarding these treatments, it is unconscionable to make such exaggerated claims about expensive products to vulnerable patients. Furthermore, patients are often led to believe that the

We would simply advise caution when seeking alternative therapies.

Other Therapies

failure of a product was due to their lack of effort or belief in the product, and that with only more effort or belief (and of course expense) benefit may arise.

93. What are clinical trials?

Clinical trials are the mechanism by which new and safer treatments are evaluated. They aim to determine whether a treatment is effective, whether it is better than existing treatments, and whether the treatment can be administered safely. It is only through carefully performed clinical trials that potential new treatments can be transferred from the laboratory to the bedside.

In the development of a new drug, "preclinical studies" are the first step. These are studies performed in laboratories and/or animals (usually mice) that provide the first indication that the drug has some activity directed against a cancer. If a drug appears promising, a phase 1 study may be performed, which is primarily conducted to determine the correct dose of the new treatment and to obtain further information about side effects. Most phase 1 studies are designed to start off at a very low dose of the medication in small groups of patients. The patients are monitored closely for the development of any side effects. If no side effects are seen, another small group of patients will be treated at a higher dose. In this fashion, subsequent patients receive increasing doses of the drug, assuming that the patients treated at the lower dose levels tolerated the medication without unacceptable side effects. In this way, the effect of the drug in humans can be assessed in a relatively safe manner. Of course, there are risks to participating in a phase 1 trial. Although unexpected side effects may exist, the possibility of obtaining a significant benefit also has potential. Often it is patients whose cancer is progressing in spite of previous treatments that are most willing to participate in phase 1 clinical trials.

After completing phase 1, new treatments enter phase 2 studies. Now that the correct dose and side effects are known, the phase 2 study is to establish that a treatment is effective. A phase 2 study involves a larger group of patients who all generally receive the same dose. They are evaluated to determine how the cancer responds to the treatment and also to gather further information about side effects.

If the treatment still appears promising, it will continue into phase 3, which is usually designed to compare the new treatment with other currently available treatments. This phase often involves a randomized study in which patients have a one in two chance of receiving the new treatment. Patients are then followed closely, and the response of patients in the two groups is compared. It is preferable that neither the patient nor his or her physician is aware of which treatment is administered, as this could lead to bias in favor of one treatment over another. A phase 3 study is the best method for demonstrating that one treatment is better than another. The Food and Drug Administration has a mandate to regulate medications. Before approval for use, all clinical trial data are reviewed to ensure that a drug meets the standards for being safe and effective.

Only through clinical trials can patients and their doctors know which treatments are best for their type of cancer. A new treatment gets evaluated because there are indications that it may be more effective, safer, or easier on the patient than an alternative treatment. Drugs that do not show promise are not further evalu-

Other Therapies

ated. If clinical trials were not conducted, physicians would have nothing concrete to guide them when making recommendations to patients. Treatments currently used for lymphoma are the direct result of previous patients volunteering for clinical trials. The dramatic improvements in survival seen among patients with Hodgkin's disease and children with leukemia are direct results of clinical trials that sequentially incorporate advances from earlier studies into subsequent studies.

Patients entering on a clinical trial are not "guinea pigs."

Patients entering on a clinical trial are not "guinea pigs." Before a clinical trial can enroll patients, it is carefully reviewed from scientific, safety, and ethical viewpoints. Patients also need to provide "informed consent," which establishes that they understand the reason for the study, the risks and possible benefits, and the availability of alternative treatment options. Institutional review boards are required to approve and monitor the conduct of clinical trials and have the ability to suspend or close a trial if there are concerns about safety.

A drug company with an interest in developing a particular drug may sponsor a clinical trial, or the funding may come from an independent source such as a university grant or a governmental agency. The same strict requirements need to be followed regardless of the source of funding.

94. Should I enter a clinical trial?

Participation in a clinical trial can be beneficial in many respects. Discuss with your lymphoma doctor whether any suitable clinical trials are available, as they often offer a way for receiving new and innovative treatments that otherwise may be unavailable.

Cancer centers often have a number of clinical trials available for different cancers. Smaller oncology practices, however, may have few or no trials available. Participation in a trial may then require travel away from home and loved ones. Because a clinical trial cannot offer any guarantee of benefit, the disruption and inconvenience may outweigh the benefit and can also be a significant emotional and financial burden for you and your family.

When deciding on participation in a clinical trial, collect as much information as possible. Find out what the treatment involves, how it is different from standard treatments, and what the relative risks and benefits are. Ask whether any other clinical trials are available and what the experience has been to date. Enquire whether the trial is phase I, phase II, or phase III, and ask what question the trial is hoping to answer.

Collect as much information as possible when deciding to participate in a clinical trial.

Before making a final decision, ensure that you have a very good understanding of the treatment involved and also of the time commitment. Find out whether there are any costs for which you are responsible. Also, try to develop an understanding of the likelihood of benefit from the treatment. Often, participating in a clinical trial is the right decision; especially at times where few other options are available, patients are vulnerable to and may reach out toward anything offering a glimmer of hope. Thoughtful discussion with your physician and sometimes a second opinion may help you to make a rational decision.

Other Therapies

95. How do I find out what clinical trials are available?

Most patients receive information about treatment options from their lymphoma physician. However, you can also find out about clinical trials from the National Cancer Institute. They can be contacted at 1–800–422–6237 or on their web site at www.cancer-trials.nci.nih.gov. Other web sites with helpful information are included in the Appendix.

PART SEVEN

Coping with Lymphoma

Can I continue to work?

Should I join a support group?

If I am dying, how do I cope?

More...

96. Can I continue to work?

Your ability to continue working will depend on your strength and endurance and also on the schedule and demands of treatment. Some patients feel well, treating lymphoma and its treatment as a minor inconvenience. They may come in for chemotherapy and then head straight to the office. Most patients, however, feel more significantly impaired and may require much rest during the day. Whether you continue to work depends on how you are feeling.

Whether you continue to work depends on how you are feeling.

Regardless, discuss your diagnosis with your employer, because you will need to take time off for medical appointments and treatments. Your employer will be much more understanding if he or she is aware of the reasons for your absence.

If you decide to not work, it's a good idea to contact your employer's human resources department, as they can inform you of the steps necessary to ensure that your medical insurance is not interrupted. You may also benefit from talking to a social worker about your eligibility for disability benefits.

97. Should I join a support group?

Support groups, which are available in most communities, may be designed for all cancer patients or for only lymphoma patients. Support groups are usually held monthly, and family members are generally welcome to attend. A support group may also be available specifically for family members.

Your attendance at a support group does not necessarily require that you open up to the group, because you may simply prefer to listen. Often it is comforting to hear the stories of how others cope with a similar illness, and you may gain some very helpful insights. If you are unsure whether you will benefit from attendance, try it once or twice, as there is no obligation to continue. Remember, however, that you may also be able to provide much comfort, support, inspiration, and advice to others in the group, especially if you continue to do well. For contact information, ask your physician or nurse or call the American Cancer Society.

98. If I am dying, how do I cope?

Because coming to terms with one's death is very difficult for most of us, advanced preparations can help. Honesty and openness with loved ones and friends are very important. Honest communication between the medical team and the patient is also very important. Death is a difficult subject for most of us to discuss, and this is certainly true of most physicians, even oncology and hematology physicians. Too frequently, this subject will not be adequately discussed, sometimes resulting in a sense of mistrust and suspicion between patients and their family members and physicians. It is very important that up-front discussions be held regarding the appropriateness of further treatment when it is unlikely to provide benefit. Patients may wish to continue treatment, even with little hope of any meaningful response. Having the ability to accept that further treatment is unlikely to be beneficial and may actually be harmful is a great step forward in accepting death. Trust in your physician is essential in reaching this realization. Even if further treatment is not physically harmful, it can deprive you of meaningful quality of life. Accepting that further treatment

You may simply prefer to listen.

Coping with Lymphoma

is futile can actually be a very empowering time. It can remove much stress and allow you to dedicate your remaining time to those who are most important to you. You may feel physically much better as further side effects of treatment are avoided. Talking to a minister or social worker can also be helpful.

Once the decision is made not to pursue further active treatment against the lymphoma, hospice may be appropriate. The hospice movement, in which the emphasis is on quality of life and symptom and pain management rather than the length of life has evolved greatly over the past 100 years. Most hospice facilities provide support to patients in their own home as much as possible.

Advance directive

a legal document that clarifies a patient's wishes in advance in the event he or she is unable to make decisions at a later time and allows the assignment of an alternative individual to make such decisions.

Durable power of attorney

a document allowing another person, usually a close relative, to make financial and medical decisions in the event that you are incapacitated.

Do not resuscitate

a state whereby aggressive life-saving measures such as cardiopulmonary resuscitation (CPR) will not be undertaken because it is unlikely to prolong useful life.

Advance planning for serious illness includes an **advance directive** and a **durable power of attorney**. An advance directive is a document that states your preferences for treatments that you will or will not accept if you are in a position in which you are unable to make such a decision. This may be the only way the medical team knows and can honor your wishes. Advance directive forms are available from your healthcare facility. An advance directive may cover such issues as a **"do not resuscitate"** order, which addresses your wishes concerning resuscitation in the event of heart or lung failure. Because resuscitation usually involves life-support apparatus, your decision about this should be made in advance.

A durable power of attorney or a healthcare proxy allows a specific family member to make decisions about your health care in the event that you are incapacitated. The durable power of attorney also allows an individual to make financial and legal decisions.

99. What happens if I have no insurance?

Patients without insurance (or even with insurance) must carry a significant financial burden because of their illness. The hospital or clinic will tell you to whom you should speak regarding financial options. Most healthcare facilities will have a financial case-worker or social worker to direct you toward some help. Government programs, disability benefits, or volunteer organizations may provide helpful resources.

The American Cancer Society has a list of useful resources on their web site (www.cancer.org) that include information regarding Medicaid and Medicare eligibility and make the following recommendations regarding dealings with your insurance company:

- Become familiar with your individual insurance plan and its provisions. If you think that you might need additional insurance, ask your insurance carrier whether it is available.
- Submit claims for all medical expenses even when you are uncertain about your coverage.
- Keep accurate and complete records of claims submitted, pending, and paid.
- Keep copies of all paperwork related to your claims, such as letters of medical necessity, bills, receipts, requests for sick leave, and correspondence with insurance companies.
- Get a caseworker, a hospital financial counselor, or a social worker to help you if your finances are limited. Often, companies or hospitals can work with you to make acceptable payment arrangements if you make them aware of your situation.
- Submit your bills as you receive them. If you become overwhelmed with bills, get help. Contact

local support organizations, such as your American Cancer Society or your state's government agencies, for additional assistance.

• Do not allow your medical insurance to expire. Pay premiums in full and on time, as it is often difficult to get new insurance.

100. Where can I find more information?

This book has only lightly discussed the information that is available to patients with lymphoma. Many resources are available through web sites of organizations that are dedicated to cancer and lymphoma. A partial list is included in the Appendix.

Organizations

The American Cancer Society
American Cancer Society National Home Office
1599 Clifton Road
Atlanta, GA 30329
Phone: 800-ACS–2345
Web site: www.cancer.org

American Society of Clinical Oncology
1900 Duke Street, Suite 200
Alexandria, VA 22314
Phone: 703–299–0150
Fax: 703–299–1044
www.asco.org

American Society of Hematology
1900 M Street NW, Suite 200
Washington DC 20036
Phone: 202–776–0544
Fax: 202–776–0545
Web site: www.hematology.org

Blood and Marrow Transplant Information Network
2900 Skokie Valley Road, Suite B
Highland Park, IL 60035
888–597–7674 or 847–433–3313
Web site: www.bmtinfonet.org

The Bone Marrow Foundation
70 East 55th Street, 20th floor
New York, NY 10022
Phone: 800–365–1336
Web site: www.bonemarrow.org

Cancer Care, Inc.
275 7th Avenue
New York, NY 10001
Phone: 212–712–8400 (administration); 212–712–8080 (services)
Web site: www.cancercare.org

Cancer Research Institute
681 Fifth Avenue
New York, NY 10022
Phone: 800–99-CANCER (800–992–26237)
Web site: www.cancerresearch.org

Cure for Lymphoma Foundation
215 Lexington Ave, 11th Floor
New York, NY 10016
Phone: 800–235–6848 or 212 213–9595
Web site: www.cfl.org

Department of Veterans Affairs
Veterans Health Association
810 Vermont Avenue, NW
Washington, DC 20420
Phone: 202–273–5400 (Washington, D.C. office)
800–827–1000 (local VA office)
Web site: www.va.gov

International Bone Marrow Transplant Registry (BMTR)
Medical College of Wisconsin
PO Box 26509
Milwaukee, WI 53226
Phone: 414–456–8325
Web site: www.ibmtr.org

Leukemia & Lymphoma Society of America
Phone: 800–955–4572 for local chapter information
Web site: www.leukemia-lymphoma.org

Lymphoma Research Foundation
111 Broadway, 19th floor
New York, NY 10006
Phone: 212–349–2910 or 800–235–6848
or
8800 Venice Boulevard, Suite 207
Los Angeles, CA 90034
Phone: 310–204–7040 or 800–500–9976
Web site: www.lymphoma.org

National Cancer Institute
National Cancer Institute Public Information Office
Building 31, Room 10A31
31 Center Drive, MSC 2580
Bethesda, MD 20892–2580
Phone: 301–435–3848 (public information office line)
Web site: www.nci.nih.gov
For Clinical Trial Information
www.nci.nih.gov/clinical_trials

National Center for Complementary and Alternative Medicine
NCCAM Clearinghouse
P.O. Box 7923
Gaithersburg, MD 20898
Phone: 888–644–6226
Web site: www.nccam.nih.gov

National Coalition for Cancer Survivorship
1010 Wayne Avenue, Suite 770
Silver Spring, MD 20910
Phone: 301–650–9127
Web site: www.cansearch.org

National Comprehensive Cancer Network
50 Huntingdon Pike, Suite 200
Rockledge PA 19046
Phone: 888–909–NCCN (888–909–6226)
Web site: www.nccn.org

Appendix

National Marrow Donor Program (NMDP)
3001 Broadway St NE, Suite 500
Minneapolis, MN 55413
Phone: 800–654–1247 or 612–627–5800
Office of Patient Advocacy
Phone: 888–999–6743
Web site: www.marrow.org

Oncology Nursing Society
501 Holiday Drive
Pittsburgh, PA 15220
Phone: 412–921–7373
Web site: www.ons.org

Social Security Administration
Office of Public Inquiries
Social Security Administration
Office of Public Inquiries
6401 Security Boulevard, Room 4-C–5 Annex
Baltimore, MD 21235–6401
Phone: 800–772–1213 or 800–325–0778 (TTY)
Web site: www.ssa.gov

United Seniors Health Cooperative (USHC)
USHC, Suite 200
409 Third Street, SW
Washington, DC 20024
202–479–6973
Phone: 800–637–2604
Web site: www.unitedseniorshealth.org

The Wellness Community
8044 Montgomery Road, Suite 170
Cincinnati, OH, 45236
Phone: 888–793-WELL
Web site: www.cancer-support.org

Well Spouse Foundation
30 E. 40th Street
New York, NY 10016
Phone: 800–838–0879 or 212–685–8815
Web site: www.wellspouse.org

Additional Web Sites with Lymphoma Information

People Living With Cancer
An ASCO web site
www.plwc.org

Lymphoma Information Network
www.lymphomainfo.net

Lymphoma Education Network
www.healthtalk.com/len

Association of Cancer Online Resources
www.acor.org

Other Web Sites of Interest

www.cancersupportivecare.com/pharmacy.html
This site covers chemotherapy drugs and ways of coping with
their side effects. It also has links to the financial assistance
programs of pharmaceutical companies.

www.usda.gov/cnpp/
The U.S. Department of Agriculture; Center for Nutrition Policy
and Promotion. This web site focuses on healthy eating habits

www.aicr.org
The American Institute for Cancer Research
This site discusses methods to reduce the risk of cancer.

www.dol.gov
Information on the Family and Medical Leave Act can be found
here.

www.cms.hhs.gov
This is the web site for the Centers for Medicare and Medicaid
Services.

www.needymeds.com
This is an information site for patient financial assistance programs for medications.

Glossary

Acquired immunodeficiency syndrome (AIDS): the syndrome resulting from infection with the human immunodeficiency virus (HIV).

Acute lymphoblastic leukemia: a fast-growing type of leukemia.

Advance directive: a legal document that clarifies a patient's wishes in advance in the event they are unable to make decisions at a later time and allows the assignment of an alternative individual to make such decisions.

Albumin: a special type of protein found in the bloodstream.

Alkylating agents: a class of chemotherapy drugs.

Allogeneic transplant: a transplant using another individual as the donor.

Alopecia: hair loss.

Alternative therapy: a therapy other than a conventionally accepted medical treatment.

Anaplastic large B cell lymphoma: a type of intermediate grade lymphoma

Anemia: a low hemoglobin level.

Anemia of chronic disease: an anemia caused by the bone marrow's reaction to being sick.

Ann Arbor Staging System: used to describe the areas in the body affected by the lymphoma. It was created at a conference held in Ann Arbor, Michigan.

Anorexia: loss of appetite.

Antibodies: specialized proteins of the immune system that help fight infections. They can also be created to recognize proteins on cancer cells as in some types of lymphoma treatments.

Antibody therapy: the use of antibodies to treat cancer.

Antiemetic: a medication to prevent nausea and vomiting.

Antigen: any substance that can induce an immune response. This could be an infection or a cancer cell.

Antitumor antibiotics: a class of chemotherapy drugs.

Aorta: the main blood vessel (artery) that carries blood from the heart to the smaller arteries delivering blood to all parts of the body.

Aplasia: a condition where blood cells are not produced.

Apoptosis: a process by which normal cells die. Some cancer cells do not die, and a failure of cells to undergo apoptosis can contribute to the growth of cancer. It is often referred to as "programmed cell death."

Arteries: the vessels that carry blood containing oxygen to the organs and tissues of the body.

Autoimmune disease: an illness in which the person's own immune system can recognize parts of its own body as foreign.

Autologous stem cell transplant: a transplant in which you are your own bone marrow stem cell donor.

B cells: a type of lymphocyte.

B symptoms: fevers, night sweats, and weight loss that may occur in lymphoma patients. They can occur individually or together.

Bacteria: one class of infectious agents.

BCNU pneumonitis: inflammation of the lungs caused by the chemotherapy drug BCNU.

Benign: a growth that is not cancerous.

Biologic therapy: treatment that focuses the body's immune system on diseased cells.

Biopsy: the removal of tissue or a fluid sample for microscopic examination.

Bolus: a rapid intravenous injection.

Bone marrow: soft substance inside many bones in the body where the blood cells are produced.

Broviac catheter: a type of catheter that goes directly into a large vein to allow easier administration of medications and blood tests.

Burkitt's lymphoma: a very rapidly growing and aggressive type of lymphoma.

CD20: a protein on the surface of B lymphocytes and most B cell lymphomas.

Cellular immune response: the part of the immune response that uses lymphocytes to directly remove antigens. In contrast, the humoral immune response uses antibodies to remove antigens.

Central nervous system: the brain and spinal cord.

Chemotherapy: treating a disease with drugs; the different types of drugs used to treat cancer.

Chronic lymphocytic leukemia: the most common slow-growing type of leukemia.

Clinical trials: research studies evaluating promising new treatments in patients.

CNOP: a combination chemotherapy regimen.

Complementary therapy: therapies used in conjunction with traditional medical treatments.

Complete blood count: a blood test looking at the red cell count, the hemoglobin, the white count, and the platelet count.

Computed tomography (CT scan): a specialized type of x-ray that creates a detailed cross-sectional view of the body.

Contrast dye: a chemical that is injected for certain x-rays, including CT scans and MRI scans, that results in better contrast pictures.

Cyclophosphamide, doxorubicin, vincristine, prednisone (CHOP): the 4 drugs that are most commonly used together to treat lymphoma.

Cytokines: chemicals produced by T-lymphocytes to generate an immune response.

Cytoplasm: the part of a cell that surrounds the central nucleus.

Dehydration: low fluids in the body, which can cause dizziness, fatigue, fainting, and other minor symptoms. If not corrected, dehydration can cause more serious problems.

Depression: a disorder characterized by excessive sadness and feelings of hopelessness.

Diaphragm: the large muscle that separates the lungs from the abdomen. Its movement is important for breathing.

Diffuse large B cell lymphoma: a type of intermediate grade lymphoma.

Dimples of Venus: the dimples seen on the skin over the sacrum on the lower back.

DNA deoxyribonucleic acid: the material that carries the genetic code for each organism or person.

Do not resuscitate: a state whereby aggressive life-saving measures, such as cardiopulmonary resuscitation (CPR), will not be undertaken because they are unlikely to prolong useful life.

Durable power of attorney: a document allowing another person, usually a close relative, to make financial and medical decisions in the event that you are incapacitated.

Endoscopy: a procedure to examine the gut with a fibreoptic light.

Enzymes: chemical messengers within the body.

Eosinophils: a type of white blood cell.

Epstein-Barr virus: the virus that causes infectious mononucleosis and can cause lymphocytes to grow abnormally.

Erythropoietin: a hormone produced by the kidneys that stimulates the bone marrow to produce red blood cells.

Esophagitis: inflammation of the esophagus.

Esophagus: the tube connecting the throat to the stomach.

Fatigue: tiredness, particularly the debilitating, continuous tiredness that signals illness or disease.

Femur: the thigh bone.

Fibrosis: the replacement of normal tissue with scar tissue.

Fine needle aspiration: a procedure to obtain a sample of tissue using a small needle.

Flow cytometry: a procedure for examining the proteins present on the surface of cells.

Follicles: round structures containing lymphocytes.

Follicular lymphomas: lymphomas composed of lymphocytes organized into round structures.

Follicular mixed small cleaved and large cell lymphoma: a follicular lymphoma with follicles containing both small and large lymphocytes.

Follicular small cleaved cell lymphoma: a follicular lymphoma with follicles containing only small cells with clefts in their nuclei.

Gallium scan: a nuclear medicine test that uses gallium to show areas of lymphoma within the body.

Gamma camera: a nuclear imaging camera that can detect radioactivity.

Gastrointestinal tract: the gut, from mouth to anus.

Graft versus host disease: an illness caused by the donor's immune system recognizing and attacking tissues and organs of the marrow recipient.

Graft versus lymphoma: a situation in which the donor's immune system recognizes the recipient's lymphoma cells as foreign and works to eliminate the lymphoma.

Granules: small particles containing enzymes.

Growth factors: chemicals that can be injected to stimulate the production of blood cells.

Hashimoto's thyroiditis: a type of inflammation of the thyroid due to abnormal recognition of the thyroid gland as foreign.

Hematocrit: a measure of the number of red cells, useful for anemia or polycythemia (too many red cells).

Hematologist/oncologist: a physician specializing in the treatment of blood disorders and cancer.

Hematology: the study of diseases of the blood, including blood cancers.

Hematopoietic stem cell: the most immature cell that develops into red cells, white blood cells, and platelets.

Hemoglobin: a protein present in red blood cells that carries oxygen.

Hepatitis C virus: one of the viruses that can infect the liver and cause chronic liver inflammation.

Hickman catheter: an intravenous line that passes through the skin into a large vein near the heart. It provides a safer and easier way to administer chemotherapy and obtain blood samples.

Hodgkin's disease: a type of lymphoma.

Human immunodeficiency virus (HIV): a virus that attacks the human immune system, leaving the carrier prone to infections.

Human leukocyte antigen typing: testing of the transplantation antigens to determine whether two people are compatible for transplantation.

Human T-cell lymphotropic virus type 1: a virus that can cause leukemia by infecting T lymphocytes

Humerus: the major bone connecting the shoulder to the elbow.

Humoral immune response: an immune response that uses antibodies rather than cells to destroy an antigen (foreign protein).

Hyperviscosity: a condition in which the blood is too thick.

Idiotype: a protein sequence on the surface of B lymphocytes that is like a fingerprint. All related lymphocytes contain the same protein sequence.

Immune molecules: chemicals involved in the mounting of an immune response.

Immune system: the complex system by which the body protects itself from harmful outside invaders.

Immunoblastic lymphoma: an aggressive type of NHL.

Immunoglobulin M: one of the 5 different types of antibodies that are part of the immune system.

Immunotherapy: treatment aimed at controlling the immune system.

Indolent: usually slow growing.

Indwelling catheter: an intravenous catheter that can remain in place for longer periods than a few days.

Infectious mononucleosis: a viral infection caused by the Epstein-Barr virus. Also called glandular fever.

Inferior vena cava: the large vein that carries blood back toward the heart.

Institutional review board: commonly termed the IRB, a review board that research studies reviews to ensure they are safe and ethical.

Interferon therapy: a type of immune therapy.

International Prognostic Index: a system to determine the prognosis of patients with lymphoma.

Interventional radiologist: a physician who is trained in using x-rays to aid in the performance of some types of surgical procedures.

Intramuscular: an injection into the muscle.

Intrathecal: an injection into the fluid surrounding the spinal cord or brain.

Karnofsky Performance Status scale: a system to evaluate how patients do when performing normal daily activities.

Lactate dehydrogenase: an enzyme measured using a simple blood test.

Laparotomy: surgery involving an incision to look directly into the abdomen.

Leukapheresis: a procedure to remove large numbers of white blood cells from the body.

Leukopenia: a low white blood cell count.

Libido: sex drive.

Local treatment: treatment aimed at a particular area of the body. For example, radiation treatment is local, whereas chemotherapy is systemic.

Low microbial diet: a diet containing low amounts of bacteria or fungi.

Lymph fluid: the fluid that carries lymphocytes around the body.

Lymph glands: the large collections of lymphocytes present at intervals throughout the lymph system. They can get big and painful in response to an infection.

Lymph node architecture: the structure of lymph nodes when they are seen under a microscope.

Lymph nodes: another term for lymph glands.

Lymphadenopathy: enlarged lymph nodes.

Lymphangiogram: an x-ray study of lymph glands after they are injected with a dye.

Lymphatic channels: the tiny vessels that connect the lymph glands.

Lymphoblastic lymphoma: an aggressive, fast-growing type of lymphoma.

Lymphocyte predominant Hodgkin's disease: a type of Hodgkin's lymphoma.

Lymphocyte-depleted Hodgkin's disease: another type of Hodgkin's lymphoma.

Lymphocytes: the main type of cell that makes up the immune system and is the abnormal cell in lymphoma.

Lymphokines: chemicals that are produced by lymphocytes and help in coordinating the immune response.

Lymphoma: cancer of the lymphocytes.

Lymphoma classification: a system to organize the many different types of lymphoma.

Lymphomatoid granulomatosis: a rare type of lymphoma.

Lymphoplasmacytic lymphoma: the lymphoma associated with Waldenstrom's macroglobulinemia.

Magnetic resonance imaging: a technique based on the use of magnetic fields to produce images of body parts.

Malaria: an infection caused by a parasite and transmitted by mosquitoes.

Malignant: cancerous.

MALT lymphomas: a type of lymphoma that tends to involve lymph glands present in the mucosa (the lining of the gut or other organs).

Mantle cell lymphoma: an uncommon type of aggressive lymphoma.

Marginal zone lymphoma: a type of indolent lymphoma.

Mediastinal nodes: lymph nodes present in the area between the lungs.

Megakaryocytes: the bone marrow cells that produce platelets.

Megestrol acetate: a medication that can increase the appetite.

Mesenteric lymph nodes: the lymph nodes present in the abdomen tissue that anchors the bowel.

Microtubules: structures present in individual cells that are important for allowing cells to divide.

Minitransplant: a transplant in which the doses of chemotherapy or radiotherapy are reduced compared to those given for a standard transplant.

Mixed cellularity Hodgkin's disease: one of the types of Hodgkin's disease.

Monoclonal antibodies: antibodies that bind to a specific target on the surface of lymphoma or other cancer cells.

Monoclonal proteins: another term for monoclonal antibodies.

Monocytes: a type of white blood cell.

Monocytoid B-cell lymphoma: an unusual type of indolent lymphoma.

Mucosa-associated lymphoid tissue: *see* MALT lymphoma.

Mycosis fungoides: a type of lymphoma that mainly involves the skin.

Mucositis: a painful condition due to breakdown of the lining of the mouth.

Neutropenia: a low level of neutrophils

Neutrophils: the main white blood cell important for fighting infection.

Nodular sclerosing Hodgkin's disease: the most common type of Hodgkin's disease.

Nodules: *see* Follicles.

Non-Hodgkin's lymphoma: the most common type of lymphoma.

Nonmyeloablative stem cell transplant: same as mini-transplant.

Nuclear medicine: the medicine specialty that deals with using radioisotopes for obtaining body scans and for treatment.

Nucleoside analogues: a type of chemotherapy drug that targets lymphocytes.

Nucleus: the central part of the cell that contains the genetic information.

Oncology: the field of medicine that studies cancer.

Palpitations: the sensation of an irregular heartbeat.

Pathologist: a physician who makes the diagnosis of lymphoma and other cancers from evaluating biopsies and other surgical specimens under the microscope.

Performance status: the level of ability with which patients can perform their routine daily activities.

Peripheral blood stem cell transplants: a transplant using marrow stem cells that have been obtained from the blood circulation.

Peripheral neuropathy: a condition caused by damage to the nerves in the arms or legs.

PET scan: *see* Positron emission tomography.

Petechiae: pinpoint red spots that occur with low platelet counts and are due to tiny areas of bleeding into the skin.

Phagocyte: a cell that scavenges other cells.

Pheresis catheter: a large indwelling catheter placed through the skin into a large vein to allow the collection of stem cells.

Phototherapy: a type of therapy using UV light.

Plasma cells: the most mature type of B cell. They produce immuno-globulins and are the malignant cell in multiple myeloma.

Plasmablastic lymphoma: a rare type of lymphoma due to immature plasma cells.

Plasmapheresis: a treatment that consists of removing plasma.

Platelets: the tiny blood cells that are produced in the bone marrow and are important for blood clotting.

Pneumocystis carinii pneumoniae: an infection affecting the lungs that can occur in people with an abnormal immune system.

Portacath: an indwelling intravenous catheter that is placed entirely under-neath the skin.

Positron emission Tomography (PET): x-ray studies that use the abnormal sugar metabolism of cancer cells to identify metastatic deposits.

Posttransplant lymphoproliferative disorders: a type of lymphoma that occurs after a transplant, usually because the immune system is depressed.

Power of attorney: *see* Durable power of attorney.

Prognosis: a prediction of the course that a disease will take.

Pulmonary function tests: a set of tests performed to evaluate the ability of the lungs to function properly.

Purging: the technique whereby certain cells (usually cancerous) are removed from the remaining cells present in the collected bone marrow or stem cells.

Radiation therapy: treatment using radiation.

Raynaud's syndrome: a disorder associated with pain and a change in color in the fingers.

Red blood cells: the most common type of blood cells that carry oxygen around the body.

Reproductive system: the body parts associated with reproduction.

Retroperitoneal lymph nodes: the most common lymph nodes present in the abdomen.

Revised European American Lymphoma classification: the basis of the newest lymphoma classification.

Rheumatoid arthritis: an autoimmune disorder associated with destruction and deformity of joints.

Saliva: the lubricating substance produced by the salivary glands that is essential for chewing and swallowing.

Salivary glands: the gland that produces saliva.

Shingles: a painful condition with a rash, usually affecting one area of the skin in the distribution of a nerve. It is due to reactivation of the chicken pox virus and usually occurs when the immune system is depressed.

Simulation: the planning necessary before administering any radiation treatment.

Sjogren's syndrome: a condition due to dryness of the eyes and mouth.

Small lymphocytic lymphoma: a type of indolent lymphoma that is similar to chronic lymphocytic leukemia.

Small noncleaved cell lymphoma: an aggressive, rapidly growing lymphoma.

Spinal fluid: the fluid surrounding the brain and spinal fluid.

Spinal tap: the procedure for obtaining a sample of spinal fluid.

Spleen: the large lymph-node–like organ under the lower left ribs.

Sporadic Burkitt's: the form of Burkitt's lymphoma that occurs in the United States.

Stage: a reference to the number of places in the body affected by lymphoma or other cancer.

Stem cell mobilization: the process by which bone marrow stem cells are stimulated to move into blood circulation.

Stem cell transplantation: the procedure of replacing bone marrow stem cells to allow recovery of blood cells after high-dose chemotherapy.

Stem cells: the cells that can produce red cells, white cells, and platelets.

Subcutaneous: underneath the skin.

Superior vena cava syndrome: a condition in which the blood flow back to the heart is decreased due to obstruction, usually by very big lymph nodes.

Systemic lupus erythematosus: a disease in which the immune system attacks the body.

Systemic treatment: a treatment, such as chemotherapy, that reaches all body parts through the bloodstream.

T cells: one of the major types of lymphocytes.

T-cell–rich B-cell lymphoma: a type of aggressive lymphoma.

Testosterone: a male hormone.

Thrombocytopenia: a low platelet count.

Thymus: an organ behind the breast bone that is important for the development of an immune response, especially in children.

Tissues: a collection of cells of a similar type with a similar function.

Tonsils: large lymph nodes present in the back of the throat.

Total body irradiation: radiation therapy administered to the entire body, usually in preparation for a transplant.

Trachea: the windpipe.

Translocation: an abnormality of certain chromosomes seen in some cancer cells.

Vaccines: an injection given to stimulate an immune response.

Veins: blood vessels that return blood to the heart.

Villi: tiny outcrops of the lining of organs, especially the bowel.

Vinca alkaloids: a type of chemotherapy drug.

Viruses: tiny infectious agents that require other cells for their growth and survival.

Waldenstrom's macroglobulinemia: a type of lymphoma that produces too much IgM and can be associated with an increased viscosity.

White blood cells: blood cells that are most important for fighting infection.

Working Formulation: one of the lymphoma classifications.

Xerostomia: dryness of the mouth due to disease.

Index